Advance Praise for *Dimension*
Problems

This book brings together Lahey's clinical acumen, commitment to evidence-based public health, and methodological sophistication to fashion a new way of thinking about psychological problems. It's an eye-opener, and a game changer. It's also a great read!

Avshalom Caspi, PhD
Edward M. Arnett Professor
Department of Psychology and Neuroscience
Duke University

Professor Lahey has written a bold and prescient book that points the way to how psychological problems will be understood and classified in the foreseeable future. For too long, these problems have been classified based on tradition, as opposed to evidence. Lahey shows how the classification of psychological problems can be based on data pointing to underlying dimensions of human experience, thereby solving numerous scientific dilemmas, while also reducing stigma. Essential reading for all practitioners, researchers, and policymakers in the field of mental health.

Robert F. Krueger, PhD
Hathaway Distinguished Professor
Distinguished McKnight University Professor
Department of Psychology
University of Minnesota

Psychological problems touch everyone. If you have ever wondered why psychological problems are diagnosed the way they are, this book is for you. Dr. Lahey explains his radical plan for how it can be done 100% better. This book needs to be heard, and if we listen, everyone's mental health will improve. The book is authoritative, it's reader-friendly, and it's very, very brave.

Terrie E. Moffitt, PhD
Nannerl O. Keohane University Distinguished Professor
Department of Psychology and Neuroscience
Duke University

A fascinating read with a bold vision that may fundamentally change how the reader will think about etiology and diagnosis. It will draw you in like a crime novel even though the first chapter gives away one culprit: the current failed psychiatric concepts. Lahey's erudite but highly accessible book offers many novel insights on the genetic structure, individual dispositions, the environmental contribution to and the hierarchy of psychological problems. There is no other book that marries our insights on the nature with those on the nurture of psychological problems so expertly and brilliantly.

Henning Tiemeier, MD, PhD
Sumner and Esther Feldberg Chair of Maternal and Child Health
Harvard University School of Public Health
Professor of Psychiatric Epidemiology
Erasmus University Medical Center

Ben Lahey puts all his years of experience into this book which is so refreshingly and eloquently written that it will inspire those who seek to expand their understanding of psychological problems. Lahey unties the chains of restricted categorical thinking and reconsiders the nature and causes of psychological problems from a dimensional perspective in a way that will renew our insights.

Frank C. Verhulst, MD, PhD
Research Professor at Erasmus University Medical Center

Dimensions of Psychological Problems

Replacing Diagnostic Categories with a More Science-Based and Less Stigmatizing Alternative

BENJAMIN B. LAHEY

*Irving B. Harris Professor of Epidemiology,
Psychiatry and Behavioral Neuroscience
Department of Public Health Sciences
University of Chicago*

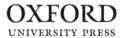

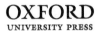

OXFORD
UNIVERSITY PRESS

Oxford University Press is a department of the University of Oxford. It furthers the University's objective of excellence in research, scholarship, and education by publishing worldwide. Oxford is a registered trade mark of Oxford University Press in the UK and certain other countries.

Published in the United States of America by Oxford University Press
198 Madison Avenue, New York, NY 10016, United States of America.

© Oxford University Press 2021

All rights reserved. No part of this publication may be reproduced, stored in a retrieval system, or transmitted, in any form or by any means, without the prior permission in writing of Oxford University Press, or as expressly permitted by law, by license, or under terms agreed with the appropriate reproduction rights organization. Inquiries concerning reproduction outside the scope of the above should be sent to the Rights Department, Oxford University Press, at the address above.

You must not circulate this work in any other form and you must impose this same condition on any acquirer.

Library of Congress Cataloging-in-Publication Data
Names: Lahey, Benjamin B., author.
Title: Dimensions of psychological problems : replacing diagnostic categories with a more science-based and less stigmatizing alternative / Benjamin B. Lahey.
Description: New York, NY : Oxford University Press, [2021] |
Includes bibliographical references and index.
Identifiers: LCCN 2021015167 (print) | LCCN 2021015168 (ebook) |
ISBN 9780197607909 (paperback) | ISBN 9780197607923 (epub) |
ISBN 9780197607930 (online)
Subjects: MESH: Diagnostic and statistical manual of mental disorders. 5th ed. |
Mental Disorders—etiology | Adaptation, Psychological |
International Classification of Diseases | Social Factors
Classification: LCC RC454 (print) | LCC RC454 (ebook) | NLM WM 31 |
DDC 616.89—dc23
LC record available at https://lccn.loc.gov/2021015167
LC ebook record available at https://lccn.loc.gov/2021015168

DOI: 10.1093/med/9780197607909.001.0001

This material is not intended to be, and should not be considered, a substitute for medical or other professional advice. Treatment for the conditions described in this material is highly dependent on the individual circumstances. And, while this material is designed to offer accurate information with respect to the subject matter covered and to be current as of the time it was written, research and knowledge about medical and health issues is constantly evolving and dose schedules for medications are being revised continually, with new side effects recognized and accounted for regularly. Readers must therefore always check the product information and clinical procedures with the most up-to-date published product information and data sheets provided by the manufacturers and the most recent codes of conduct and safety regulation. The publisher and the authors make no representations or warranties to readers, express or implied, as to the accuracy or completeness of this material. Without limiting the foregoing, the publisher and the authors make no representations or warranties as to the accuracy or efficacy of the drug dosages mentioned in the material. The authors and the publisher do not accept, and expressly disclaim, any responsibility for any liability, loss, or risk that may be claimed or incurred as a consequence of the use and/or application of any of the contents of this material.

3 5 7 9 8 6 4 2

Printed by Marquis, Canada

Contents

Foreword   vii
    Stephen P. Hinshaw
Preface   xv
Acknowledgments   xix

1. Conceptualizing Psychological Problems   1

2. From Binary Diagnostic Categories to Dimensions
   of Psychological Problems   29

3. Dimensions of Internalizing Problems   53

4. Dimensions of Externalizing Problems   68

5. Dimensions of Psychotic and Other Problems
   of Thought and Affect   95

6. Hierarchical Nature of Psychological Problems   113

7. Sex Differences and the Dynamic Development of
   Psychological Problems   135

8. Ordinary Origins of Psychological Problems:
   Genetic–Environmental Interplay   164

9. Ordinary Origins of Psychological Problems:
   Transacting with the World   187

Epilogue   215
Technical Appendix   219
Index   225

Foreword

Just what *is* mental disorder—or as it's often termed in medical literature, mental illness? This seemingly basic question has plagued philosophy, religion, science, and clinical practice for millennia.

In *Dimensions of Psychological Problems*, Benjamin Lahey expounds
upon a radically simple model related to ordinary processes in development. He contends that what we commonly term mental disorders
are in fact *not* actual disease states but instead the extremes of
distributions along several underlying and fairly universal dimensions
of thought, emotion, and behavior. In other words, rather than comprising categorical "boxes" denoting qualitative, essentialist medical
conditions, these problems are actually the product of genetic liabilities and contextual processes that render some individuals—at some
points of their life spans—to experience non-normative levels of maladjustment (related to either their well-being or, for externalizing/ag-
gressive problems, injury and impairment for those with whom they
interact). In fact, nearly all of us will encounter such extremes of psychological problems during our lifetimes, often in waxing or waning
patterns. Forerunners of these issues typically emerge during childhood and adolescence, via the unfolding of transactional patterns of
risk and protective factors, featuring within-individual propensities
that work in tandem with social and economic forces.

Indeed, the sheer *ordinariness* of psychological problems (often
branded as psychopathology in scientific research) is the underlying
message of this book. But ordinary does not begin to describe the importance of the messages or the clarity of the writing. Instead, they are
both extraordinary.

Lahey argues that true mental *illnesses* do not exist, at least as a
set of categorical disease entities. Yet he makes haste to differentiate
this perspective from half-century-old notions that mental disorders
are just myths, a la Thomas Szasz. Lahey is clear that psychological

problems—especially at the extremes of relevant distributions and particularly those with early life onset—can be devastating to individuals, families, communities, and even entire societies, comprising far more than sheer problems in living. As he readily admits, many other clinical scientists are converging on these perspectives (even though Lahey is overly modest in discussing his own extensive scientific output along such lines). He thus joins such efforts as developmental psychopathology; the National Institute of Mental Health's Research Domains Criteria; and the growing number of investigators interested in hierarchical models of psychopathology, including the Hierarchical Taxonomy of Psychopathology.

Among the key features of Lahey's formulation, I begin with the core position that psychopathology is decidedly *not* "all or none." I remember vividly that as a graduate student many years back, I learned that one either had or did not have autism, or bipolar disorder, or schizophrenia, or hyperactivity [the forerunner term for attention-deficit/ hyperactivity disorder (ADHD)]. Today, massive amounts of research have revealed that nearly every form of psychological dysfunction/ psychopathology lies on a continuum with more normative patterns of behavior. Think of current terms such as autism spectrum disorders or bipolar spectrum conditions: The core subject matter is *gradations* of behavior, thought, and affect. Determining what is normative versus what is atypical entails major efforts to ascertain accurate cutoff points, just as is the case for medical conditions such as high normal versus pathologically high blood pressure. Yet in the case of behavior and emotion, making such determinations is greatly complicated by knotty problems related to self-reports (or informant reports) of problems, as opposed to objective biological indicators, along with comparisons to social and cultural standards that provide key comparisons for behavioral normality.

In many respects, Lahey's arguments are parallel to important perspectives from evolutionary psychology, which posits that what are today considered mental disorders or diseases are in fact adaptations. That is, anxiety "disorders" in modern, urban societies may represent perfectly functional alarm functions in relation to potentially threatening stimuli from earlier phases of human evolution—which become dysfunctional only in the context of contemporary, postindustrial, sedentary contexts. Similar lines of reasoning may well apply to many variants of depressive affect and behavior, which can be viewed as largely expectable responses to loss or defeat. Moreover, in relation to genetic vulnerability, what may be quite deleterious if evidenced in full form could actually be adaptive in a heterozygotic configuration (in relation to two different alleles of a certain gene)—or, at a dimensional level, less "loaded" combinations of risk alleles.

Furthermore, it goes without saying (yet still needs to be emphasized, as Lahey carefully does) that genes always interact and transact with context, epigenetically and beyond—both within individuals and across members of a species. It would be a major mistake to posit that mental disorders are inevitably the product of "bad" or maladaptive genes, if context is ignored. (Admittedly, as I highlight at the end of this Foreword, in some instances, specific genetic abnormalities do underlie serious problems of adjustment, particularly related to neurodevelopmental conditions such as autism or ADHD.) Yet it is an equal mistake to take on the wholly cultural-contextual viewpoint that what we term maladjustment is solely the product of deviance from personal standards or social norms. Doing so can conflate nonconformity, or religious/political difference, with psychological maladjustment. In the end, true integration across (a) heritable risk and (b) contextual influences that transact with such risk remains the holy grail of psychological and psychiatric research and clinical efforts.

Crucially, Lahey is an ardent advocate for the evidence-based position that we cannot rely on cross-sectional data alone. In other words, a longitudinal perspective on developmental pathways and transactional influences is essential. This book would need to transform into a multivolume set to give testimony to the myriad unfolding pathways—at the confluence of genes, temperament, attachment, later parental influences, schooling, neighborhood contexts, and community-/policy-level influences—that constitute the detailed subject matter of typical versus less typical developmental outcomes. Lahey also strongly contends that examination of differences across sex and gender is crucial for understanding the origins and continuities of psychological adjustment and maladjustment over the life course. Racial/ethnic, socioeconomic, and cultural forces must also be part of the equation.

A fundamental perspective throughout the book, as noted in its subtitle, is that a perspective embracing dimensions of psychological problems as opposed to reified categories of disease states can aid in reducing the pervasive stigmatization that still, even in our postmodern era, clings to the subject matter at hand. Much of my own thinking, writing, and research of late focuses on the topic of stigma reduction. There's no room for a thorough essay on this subject matter in a book foreword, but evidence is building that at least in some domains, when individuals come to view psychological problems as occurring on a continuum with normative behaviors/thoughts/emotions, social distance and stigmatization will lessen. Indeed, the belief that we all struggle with fluctuations in and out of maladjustment, that some of us are more vulnerable than others to heart disease or depression, and that in the end we're all human could go an extremely long way.

Even more, research syntheses reveal that when research participants are led to believe that mental disorders are solely the result of biogenetic abnormalities (e.g., being called "brain diseases"), they hold the individuals in question less blameworthy for maladaptive behavior but at the same time perceive them as relatively unchangeable and potentially more violent. This is what our Australian colleague Nick Haslam calls the "mixed blessings" model of ascribing mental disorder solely to biogenetic causes.

Of course, we do want to acknowledge biological vulnerability, in transaction with adverse experiences and environments. Eschewing biological and genetic risk completely could lead to a wrongminded retreat to views from earlier eras that psychological problems are the result of evil spirits—or more recent perspectives that they emanate from weak personal character or exclusively from maladaptive parenting. Note that the inaccurate, denigrating, and now-discounted refrigerator-parent theories of autism or the stereotype of the schizophrenogenic mother are only a few decades behind us.

In the end, beyond policy changes and dissemination efforts that can make evidence-based treatments more accessible to those with psychological issues, *humanization* is crucial. Personal and family narratives breed enhanced empathy and increased support. As in the case of cancer—a highly stigmatized illness for much of the 20th century—when it's acceptable to form solidarity with fellow fighters/

survivors and when the general public realizes that there's no shame involved, attitudes can and do change and reinvigorated scientific and clinical action will ensue. Lahey's nonsensationalized encapsulations of internalizing, externalizing, and thought problem behaviors in the book's middle chapters serve as a model of bridging typical versus less typical manifestations of these behavior patterns. Along with more explicitly personal accounts, these can promote resilience as well as family and group support.

Beyond the clarity of his language on each and every page, Lahey is admirably honest in his ability to say "I don't know . . ." about the sheer complexity of influences and processes related to psychopathology at the onset of the third decade of the 21st century. Clearly, however, he knows a lot. He also tackles a host of long-standing issues and puzzles that continue to plague scientific and clinical efforts. Comorbidity is a core example. Categorical views of mental disorder are simply unable to explain the empirical demonstration that most people experiencing a given form of mental illness often simultaneously or sequentially meet criteria for one or many more additional categories. If mental disorders were truly independent, such joint occurrences (called comorbidities) would be quite rare. Although categorical diagnostic systems cannot explain such well-beyond-chance instances of multiple disorders, dimensional perspectives readily take into account the interlinked and hierarchical nature of psychopathology from a multidimensional perspective. Furthermore, it may well be the case that what appears—spanning childhood, adolescence, and young adulthood—as a series of unfolding conditions (e.g., ADHD to oppositional defiant disorder to substance use disorder to antisocial personality disorder), the dimensional perspective, when enriched by developmental psychopathology, is in synch with the concept of *heterotypic continuity*. That is, underlying vulnerabilities, subsequently shaped by less than adaptive environmental contexts, can unleash a cascade of age-dependent manifestations of, in this instance, an underlying externalizing dimension. This is quite a different perspective from claiming that the individual in question simply graduates from one form of mental disorder to another independent form.

This book is a clear antidote to the reductionist tendencies that have plagued the field of mental health science since its inception, largely in the form of all-biology versus all-family or all-psychosocial influences. Lahey also realizes the potential for strength and personal adaptation that can emerge for many individuals who place high on various dimensions of psychological distress.

Is *Dimensions of Psychological Problems* the definitive answer regarding the nature of and mechanisms underlying psychological problems? Of course not, as Lahey himself would readily admit. Our field is simply not mature enough at the levels of scientific and theoretical understanding. Yet the book should elevate researchers and clinicians alike to a new point of fruitful debate and future directions.

Given the book's insistence that psychological problems are indeed ordinary, the reader may think that Lahey underestimates or understates the too often severe consequences of such problems. Yet he clearly acknowledges the potential for serious impairments. Even so, I take pains to highlight the relevant devastation that can be part of the mix, involving the crushing levels of despair, hopelessness, financial ruin, family disintegration, and staggering societal costs that can ensue. In fact, as now regularly reported in the media, suicide rates are growing in most (but not all) countries on earth, particularly the United States—especially for young people, particularly girls. The prevalence of mood and anxiety disorders, as well as in-home violence and child maltreatment, is clearly accentuated by the current COVID-19 pandemic, with consequences bound to ensue for years to come. The diagnosed prevalence of neurodevelopmental conditions such as ADHD and autism spectrum disorders has skyrocketed during the past two decades (whether the true prevalence is similarly expanding is another huge question). Blatant economic disparities in far too many countries have the potential for ever-growing incidence of serious psychological problems. In short, the sheer waste of human potential brought on by developmentally extreme levels of behavior, thought, and affect is staggering.

There's another potential danger that a shallow reading of the book's messages could induce. If, as noted previously, the ultimate conclusion is that the kinds of problems discussed in its pages are so ordinary as to be simple violations of social norms—without taking into account the clear evidence for transactions across heritable risk and contextual forces as the drivers of dysfunction—we could end up in the nonproductive world of the 1960s when mental illnesses were believed to be mythical, the sole artifacts of repressive political systems, or the products of faulty parenting above all else. On the other hand, we cannot abide a return to the horrific "science" and policies related to the eugenics movements of a century ago. I urge readers to read this book carefully—especially Chapters 8 and 9, in which Lahey explicitly synthesizes rather than fractionates the dual, interacting roles of genes and environments (including not just families but also schools, neighborhoods, and cultures) in shaping individual differences in key behavioral dimensions. In short, despite the supposed simplicity and ordinariness of processes underlying people's placement on behavioral dimensions, the processes involved are massively complex and still far from adequately understood. Although these chapters will be technically challenging for many readers, their inclusion of both historical and extremely recent research findings and their massively integrationist messages are essential to take in.

I suspect that in the decades to come, the field will come to the conclusion that some of the most severe psychological problems in the domain of psychopathology should actually be recognized as disease states (and perhaps migrate to the field of neurology). This is undoubtedly the case for certain individuals with, for example, autism spectrum disorders (and other neurodevelopmental conditions) in whom certain key genetic sequences are spontaneously altered via copy-number variants. In addition, neural markers and even abnormalities related to highly extreme scores on thought and mood dimensions are increasingly evident (although not yet fully predictive of individual cases), related to some individuals with what we today categorize as schizophrenia and bipolar disorder. Indeed, in medicine, although systolic and diastolic blood pressure are clearly continuous measures, certain individuals with extremely high levels show qualitative differences from the rest of the population in terms of risk factors and underlying biological mechanisms. In the main, however, most "extreme scorers" are quantitatively but not qualitatively different from those scoring lower.

Overall, I recommend *Dimensions of Psychological Problems* to a wide variety of students and trainees, clinicians of many stripes, investigators of basic biological and social forces linked to promotion of serious life adjustment problems, and clinical researchers looking for a sound grounding in dimensional approaches to psychopathology and the transactional forces underlying the tragic suffering and impairment so often linked to extreme psychological problems. Curious and ambitious general readers will also be intrigued and well educated. In the end, we simply can't afford, any longer, to promote views emphasizing either the supremacy of biology and heritability or the predominance of adverse life experiences and contextual factors, at the expense of the other. My strong prediction is that you'll come away from Lahey's integrationist perspective with an appetite whetted to dive deeper, learn more, and promote humanization as an antidote to the still-rampant stigma clinging to the variety of distressing psychological problems that comprise the subject matter of this most important book. Our future as a species depends on such understanding and on relevant research progress and social action.

Stephen P. Hinshaw
University of California, Berkeley
University of California, San Francisco
January, 2021

Preface

Human beings have adapted to life on Earth remarkably well despite our physical limitations. We're not the strongest, fastest, or the most fiercely jawed and clawed of the animal species, but as a group, we're clever and resourceful survivors. Most humans live sufficiently well-nourished lives to find mates and pass their genes to their offspring. In that sense, we're a Darwinian success story that has gone from a few early humans arising in Africa to the billions that now inhabit Earth. It's fair to say, moreover, that the human race has done far more than just survive and multiply. We've accomplished extraordinary things in art, music, literature, drama, architecture, technology, science, and mathematics.

And yet, our lives are far from perfect. Nearly all of us feel uncomfortable emotions at times—fear, worry, anger, sadness, and the like. Many of us struggle to focus on the details of important tasks that do not easily capture our attention, and large numbers of us behave in a variety of ways that are self-defeating in the long term. More than a few of us use mind-altering substances that give short-term relief at tremendous long-term costs. Some of us experience a world that is not shared with others—seeing, hearing, or believing things that others think belie logic and reality. These experiences often cause us misery and interfere with our relationships with others, our education and jobs, and put us in harm's way.

This book is written to join with other psychologists and psychiatrists in advocating a new way of thinking about psychological problems that will allow us to understand psychological problems better and minimize their impact on our lives. Many of us believe that a *positive revolution* in our understanding of psychological problems is needed that rejects key elements of the status quo view held by most psychiatrists and psychologists. This is a manifesto for that revolution, which will require several related changes in thinking: We need to affirm that there is no qualitative difference in kind between "normal" and "abnormal" psychological functioning. Rather, psychological problems are problematic ways of thinking, feeling, and behaving that lie on continuous dimensions from minor to severe. Psychological problems are not distinct categories with clear boundaries among them that have their own separate causes. Instead, the dimensions of psychological problems are correlated rather than distinct, which means that people often experience psychological problems on more than one dimension at the same time. Far from muddling our understanding of the nature and causes of psychological problems, however, viewing psychological problems as correlated dimensions reveals a hierarchy of both overlapping and unique causes of each dimension that should advance our understanding of the origins of psychological problems.

Most important, we must stop believing that psychological problems reflect rare and terrifying "illnesses" of the mind. Psychological problems are *ordinary* aspects of our lives that lie on a continuum from minor to extreme. Crucially, psychological problems are ordinary in the sense of arising through the same natural processes as all aspects of our behavior. This is true even for people who struggle with extraordinarily disabling psychological problems at the extremes of the continuum. Furthermore, psychological problems are ordinary in the sense of being far more commonplace than we usually think. I present convincing evidence from recent research that shows that the *great majority* of us will experience uncomfortable and disruptive psychological problems at some time during our lives. That statement may take your breath away, but it should not. I am most definitely *not* saying that nearly all of us will fall into an abyss of mental disease—that is the ill-conceived and harmful view of psychological problems that we must leave behind. Psychological problems do not arise when a normal mind falls apart; they are just natural aspects of the human experience. Most of us will experience distressing and disruptive psychological problems during some part of our lives that are on natural continua from minor to serious.

This book presents urgent and important reasons for rejecting the dominant model of mental health problems laid out in the current 5th edition of the *Diagnostic and Statistical Manual of Mental Disorders* (DSM), published by the American Psychiatric Association, and in the 11th edition of the *International Classification of Diseases* (ICD), published by the World Health Organization. Those diagnostic manuals are based on a broken model of psychological problems that causes us more harm than good. This book is not an "anti-psychiatry" statement in any sense, however. My opposition is not to the discipline of psychiatry but, rather, to the ways in which psychological problems are defined in the DSM. My goal is to explain a new way of thinking about psychological problems that will serve all of us better. By "all of us," I mean both those of us with psychological problems and the psychiatrists, psychologists, counselors, and social workers who do their best to help people with their problems. Many professionals are ready to give that broken model up, but because the DSM view is deeply entrenched, others will feel threatened by what I say.

Some of the important ideas behind this book were first expressed by prescient psychologists and psychiatrists more than 50 years ago, but their views failed to become the dominant way of thinking about psychological problems. Their time had not yet come. Today, however, I am one voice in a growing clamor from an international group of leading psychologists and psychiatrists who are advocating these and other new ideas. The difference is that there is now remarkable new scientific evidence that I believe is strong enough to give these ideas sufficient weight to break from outdated ways of thinking. A tipping point has been reached. Although what we don't know about psychological problems in still much greater than what we do know, the time is right to pull together what has been learned by science recently to articulate this revolutionary view of psychological problems in a way that can gain more traction than in the past.

This book on psychological problems is grounded equally in science and humanism. Psychological problems are not caused by failures of character and are not products of diseased minds. Rather, they are ordinary, if often very painful, outcomes of individual differences in *normal psychological processes*. The strongest argument for a humanistic view of psychological problems comes from the new scientific data reported here. My strong hope is that thinking about psychological problems in dimensional terms will reduce our tendency to stigmatize them in ourselves and others. It will be much more difficult to stigmatize psychological problems when we accept that almost all of us will experience them at some point in our lives. Stigma makes the lives of everyone with psychological problems markedly worse by making it difficult to seek help when it's needed, creating barriers that make adaptive functioning more difficult, and adding layers of negative feelings about our psychological problems that worsen them unnecessarily.

This book shows how we can and why we should replace the diagnostic categories of DSM and ICD with an entirely *dimensional model of psychological problems*. To a much greater extent than at any time in human history, we now have enough data to present a comprehensive description of the dimensions of psychological problems. Even so, writing such a description of the nature of psychological problems requires extrapolation from, and even speculation based on, what has been discovered by science to date. In my professional life, I have worked in the trenches of psychological research. It is time, however, for me to step aside from that role long enough to describe the big picture of psychological problems as we now understand them, even if that sometimes means making educated guesses about topics that are still understudied. I am fully aware that it is always premature to write a book like this, and I want readers to be equally aware of that fact. I will be careful to distinguish statements about human problems that are based on replicated evidence from hypotheses that go beyond the current data. If one is to pause in the midst of the ongoing work of science to write out what has been learned to date in a comprehensive narrative, this is the best one can do. This means, of course, that new data in the future could invalidate some or even most of what I write. The goal of science, after all, is to become increasingly less wrong in our understanding of nature over time.

This book is written for the educated general public and for psychologists, psychiatrists, counselors, and social workers who work in clinical practice or academia. It is particularly intended for students and residents who will be entering the helping professions because the world in which they will work is rapidly changing and they need to understand why.

Acknowledgments

I am deeply indebted to Stephen Hinshaw for commenting on early drafts of the chapters in extremely helpful ways and for writing the insightful Foreword to the book. I also most sincerely thank Howard Abikoff, Brooks Applegate, Caryn Carlson, Avshalom Caspi, Paul Frick, Estelle Higgins, Robert Krueger, Terrie Moffitt, Millicent Perkins, Henning Tiemeier, and Frank Verhulst for their often very detailed comments on the manuscript as it progressed. If this book has something useful to offer, it is largely because of their very generous efforts, trenchant challenges, and insightful suggestions.

1

Conceptualizing Psychological Problems

Human lives are generally successful and often quite wonderful, yet they are easily derailed, frequently at odds with our needs, and too often punctuated by misery. Sometimes, our woes are caused by events that are completely out of our control, such as floods, pandemics, racism, and economic injustice, but our misery and dysfunction often arise from, and are an inherent part of, our own behavior. That is the topic of this book. Psychological problems are simply aspects of our behavior—broadly defined in this book to include ways of thinking, perceiving, feeling, and acting—that cause us distress or interfere with functioning in important areas of our lives.

This straightforward and pragmatic definition of psychological problems is offered as an alternative to the current view that dominates thinking about psychological problems in the Western world today. Like a growing number of other psychologists and psychiatrists,[1-5] I have come to believe that the way that we currently view psychological problems has caused us no end of difficulties. Specifically, the current 5th edition of the *Diagnostic and Statistical Manual of Mental Disorders* (DSM-5), published by the American Psychiatric Association, and the 11th edition of the *International Classification of Diseases* (ICD), published by the World Health Organization, conceptualize psychological problems as binary categories of *mental disorders* that reflect dysfunctional mental processes within the individual that are qualitatively different from "normal" mental processes. This view of psychological problems, which I refer to as the DSM model for brevity, is deeply embedded in our everyday conceptions of psychological problems and is both misleading and dangerous. Simply put, the issue is this: The way in which we define and understand psychological problems is fundamentally important because it determines how we *think and feel* about them—and how we think and feel about psychological problems determines what we *do* about them. This book urges you to reconsider how you view psychological problems and encourages you to leave behind the DSM view of categories of mental disorders.

Human beings have tried to understand psychological problems since at least the beginnings of recorded history, and, sadly, most of our attempts to understand them have been counterproductive. Our earliest views treated people with psychological problems as if their problems were caused by gods, demons, or moral turpitude. The *medical model of psychological problems*, which became dominant in Western countries around the turn of the 19th century, brought people with psychological problems into the care of physicians rather than priests or the lay wardens of asylums. The medical model of psychological problems was spelled out 2,400 years ago by Hippocrates, who believed that psychological problems were manifestations of imbalances in the four fluids or humors of the body—blood, phlegm, black bile, and yellow bile. The medical model of psychological problems was given new life in the 1800s, however, by the truly astonishing discovery by Richard Krafft-Ebing and others that the germs that cause syphilis sometimes infect the brain, resulting in the then common debilitating syndrome of psychosis and cognitive deterioration known as general paresis. Using scientific methods that now seem crude and unethical, Krafft-Ebing vaccinated persons who displayed general paresis—who were almost certainly in no state to give informed consent to be in his experiments—with puss from syphilitic chancres. Krafft-Ebing found that they responded to the vaccinations as if they already were infected with syphilis. He correctly deduced that the syphilis infection also caused general paresis. When the successful treatment of syphilis with penicillin was perfected during World War II, the previously high number of new cases of persons entering asylums each year with general paresis fell nearly to zero in the Western world. It was an electrifying scientific triumph! Understandably, this truly remarkable advance in alleviating human suffering led to the optimistic belief that every kind of psychological problem would eventually be found to be caused by germs affecting the brain. The parallel discovery that typhoid infections sometimes cause severe psychological problems[6] only added to this optimistic view. These discoveries led to the belief that psychological problems are actually medical problems and led to the current belief that medical doctors are the professionals who should treat psychological problems.

There is, of course, every reason to provide medical treatments to persons with treatable infections that cause psychological problems. Very few other infections that cause psychological problems subsequently have been discovered, however. This fact should have led to a delimited medical model of psychological problems, but it did not. Very unfortunately, the medical model took on a much broader *metaphorical meaning* when few additional links between germs and psychological problems were discovered. The logic of the modern medical model was extended to metaphorical "diseases of the mind"— syndromes of mental "symptoms" without known biological illnesses.[7]

For some scholars who endorse this contemporary medical model, the analogical use of the term "mental illness" is justified by the expectation that the discoveries of the biological "illnesses" in the brain underlying every mental disorder will come in the future.[7] For other contemporary medical model theorists, however, the term mental illness is simply an apt metaphor in which "illnesses of the *mind*" are analogous to illnesses of the brain.[8] For them, mental illnesses are "real" whether we understand their biological basis or not. Most psychologists and psychiatrists active today were trained to believe that they can discern the difference between "normal" and "abnormal" minds and thereby "diagnose mental illnesses." This is an entirely fictional and baseless notion, however, that is toxic to people with psychological problems.

The DSM Model of Psychological Problems

The definition of mental disorder in the DSM-5 states that "a mental disorder is a syndrome characterized by clinically significant disturbance in an individual's cognition, emotional regulation, or behavior that reflects a dysfunction in the psychological, biological, or developmental processes that underlie mental and behavioral functioning" (p. 20).[9] This is a contemporary version of the analogical medical model of psychological problems. To its credit, DSM-5 no longer refers to psychological problems as mental illnesses, as was the case in the first editions of the DSM. Nonetheless, the foundations of the current DSM in the medical model are revealed in its use of the medical terms of "symptom," "diagnosis," and "psychopathology." The term psychopathology is particularly telling because it is a direct synonym for mental illness (i.e., *psycho* = "mental" and *pathology* = "illness"). Indeed, the introduction to DSM-5 explicitly posits a clear line between having a mental disorder and being normal: "It requires clinical training to recognize . . . a psychopathological condition in which physical signs and symptoms exceed normal ranges" (p. 19).[9]

As stated in the Preface, this book should not be read as an "antipsychiatry" diatribe. My opposition is not to the field of psychiatry, but to the ways in which psychological problems are conceptualized and defined in the DSM. My goal is to address key issues regarding how we think about psychological problems in the context of recent empirical evidence and to advocate a *dimensional* way of conceptualizing psychological problems that will better serve both those of us who experience psychological problems and the professionals who do their best to help people with their problems. I am just one of many voices in what is becoming a loud clamor for the kinds of changes in thinking outlined in this book. The differences between the DSM view and a dimensional approach to psychological problems are very important, and we ask you to hear us out.

I acknowledge here that I played a minor role in the fourth and fifth editions of the DSM. I was a member of the DSM-IV work group that defined the mental disorders that typically begin in childhood, and I was the director of the DSM-IV field trials for the kinds of psychological problems that I later refer to in this book as externalizing problems in children and adolescents.[10,11] In addition, I served as a consultant to the DSM-5 work group on these problems. I never accepted the medical model of mental disorders, but I saw the DSM as a necessary evil when I did that work. Because the DSM dominated thinking about psychological problems, and governed access to insurance reimbursement, I decided to use data as best as I could to guide the selection of symptoms and diagnostic thresholds. If DSM had to exist, I thought it should be based on solid empirical evidence. The big change in my thinking is that I now believe the *DSM either should no longer exist or that DSM-6 should adopt a fully dimensional model* such as the one presented in this book. Audacious proclamations such as this one should be ignored unless they are backed by sound arguments, of course. That is what I hope to accomplish in this book.

A "New" Model of Psychological Problems

This book argues that it is past time to discard the medical model of psychological problems and replace it with a simpler and more pragmatic model. In one sense, this will require a *revolution* in thinking. Moving from DSM to the thinking expressed in this book is a big change and that will be difficult for many to accept. Several key aspects of the approach advocated in this book are not new at all, however. The first and most important intellectual shots in the revolution that I advocate were fired by prescient scholars more than 50 years ago. In particular, psychologist Albert Bandura[12] pragmatically defined "abnormal behavior" without reference to mental illness simply as "behavior that is harmful to the individual or departs widely from accepted social and ethical norms" (p. 10). Psychiatrist Thomas Szasz[13] similarly advocated replacing the term of mental illness with Harry Stack Sullivan's far less judgmental phrase, *problems in living*.[14] Szasz has been widely misunderstood as denying the existence psychological problems. He explicitly did not do so, but he denied the meaningfulness of the concept of mental illnesses based on an analogy to medical illness.

Like Bandura, then, I define *psychological problems* in this book as any aspect of behavior—referring broadly to our feelings, thoughts, perceptions, motives, and actions—that is distressing or impairs our successful functioning in school, work, families, or in other important areas of life. Human beings behave in a diversity of different ways, and some of these individual differences in our behavior make us miserable and interfere with our lives. If that is the case for you, you have a psychological problem in the simple, pragmatic, and nonjudgmental sense that I am advocating. Conversely, if your ways of thinking, feeling, and behaving are working well for you, then you do not have a psychological problem. That's all there is to it. No abnormal or sick minds; just behavior that is—or is not—working for you. This is all a matter of degree, of course. There is not a natural threshold between adaptive behavior and psychological problems in DSM or in this book or anywhere else. This is because psychological problems are on a continuum with no natural dividing lines. Imagine being invited to a social gathering of people you do not know. Some of us would approach that event confidently, others with a slight frisson of nervousness, some with considerable apprehension about whether we will be liked, and others would attend the event but suffer silently during the social interactions. Some of us would be so anxious that we would turn down the invitation altogether.

Where along this continuum of social anxiety is it sensible to draw a line and say we have a *social anxiety problem*? Is the answer in the DSM? To be fair, the many professionals who contributed to DSM-5 did their level best to sensibly define how much social anxiety is required for it to be considered a mental disorder. DSM-5 diagnostic criteria were written in good faith to define a clear boundary between "normal" and "abnormal" social anxiety. Unfortunately, the DSM criteria are not only vague but also make the judgment more complicated in some ways. To meet the specific DSM diagnostic criteria for social anxiety disorder, for example, social situations must "almost always" cause intense anxiety or feelings of panic. Therefore, according to this diagnostic definition, a person who experiences intense anxiety in social situations less than half of the time but finds this unpredictable social anxiety to be so painful that they quit a good job in sales and are unemployed for 2 years would not meet DSM diagnostic criteria for social anxiety disorder—because the social anxiety does not occur "almost always." Despite the clear distress and impaired life functioning, this person would be considered not to qualify for the diagnosis of social anxiety disorder according to DSM diagnostic criteria.

The dimensional view of psychological problems presented in this book takes a very different approach. It is entirely pragmatic. The only time you need to make a dichotomous decision about your level of psychological problems is when you are deciding if you want to seek help or not. And, that is up to you. You can decide that your thoughts, feelings, and actions are distressing enough, or interfere with your life enough, to seek help *at any point* on the continuum.

In making the decision to seek help, it is prudent to consider any downsides inherent in getting help—there are financial costs to consider, some risk of entering psychotherapy with a therapist who turns out to be unqualified, and risks involved in medication and other medical treatments. But, if the distress and impaired functioning that you currently experience—and may experience in the future if you do not get help—outweigh those usually small risks, then you could consider yourself in need of help in that pragmatic sense. This approach to defining psychological problems is pleasingly simple and fully meaningful. One certainly does not have to decide that one has a *sick mind* to seek help!

Because the views of Bandura and others that are the foundation of this chapter have been around for a while, I suspect that many contemporary psychologists and psychiatrists already agree with them. They have simply gotten out of the habit of thinking about psychological problems in this way. Therefore, for a sizable portion of the professional community, the revolution I advocate will require only a reawakening. Hopefully, this book will be their nudge. It is needed because even professionals who explicitly subscribe to the pragmatic definition of psychological problems offered by Bandura have been drawn into using medical model terms and concepts on a daily basis. This is because the insurance companies that provide reimbursement to psychologists and psychiatrists for their services require us to use the medical terminology and definitions enshrined in the DSM. It may make sense from the perspective of a health insurance company only to reimburse services that treat "medical conditions," but it forces psychiatrists, psychologists, and other helping professionals to address psychological problems in medical terms. This leads all of us to think about psychological problems in genuinely harmful ways, usually without realizing that we are doing so.

If we adopt the dimensional view advocated in this book, a new strategy will be needed to provide resources for people who seek help with their psychological problems. It is easy to imagine a system that provides help to all who seek it, without requiring them to have health insurance and without subjecting themselves to a diagnosis of mental illness codified in some book. This might be politically difficult to achieve, but it would be just and would not be impractical.

Social Conflict and Psychological Problems

It is important to note that the various editions of the DSM have specifically stated that persons cannot be given the diagnosis of a mental disorder if their behavior solely reflects their conflicts with society. This rule was added to prevent psychiatrists from, for example, labeling persons who disagreed with the government about a war or other policies as "crazy." This is not a hypothetical risk as there were pressures from the Richard Nixon administration to view protestors against the Vietnam War as psychotic in the United States and the former Soviet Union locked political dissidents in mental hospitals by branding their disagreements with the government signs of mental disorder. Such efforts to consider dissidents to be mentally ill could easily arise again in the future in any country. Clearly, disagreements with society should never, by themselves, be considered to be psychological problems. That said, as discussed later in this book, many individuals whose race, ethnicity, sexual orientation, or gender identities are in the minority often are deeply distressed by the discriminatory treatment they receive from the majority. Because there is no assignment of fault in the view espoused in this book, it is perfectly legitimate for individuals to seek help for distress caused by such conflicts with society if they choose. You do not have to be considered mentally ill to seek treatment in the view expressed in this book; you just need to want assistance with your distress or impairment, no matter how it arises. This is not to say, of course, that we should not make all possible efforts to reduce all forms of discriminatory treatment of those who are in the minority. Providing professional help with the psychological effects of discrimination and maltreatment is certainly not enough. Psychological problems can be prevented by reducing discrimination and maltreatment.

Ordinariness of Psychological Problems

A key theme of this book is that psychological problems are *ordinary*. Why do I say this? I certainly do not mean that they are always minor and can be ignored; psychological experiences often make us miserable and interfere significantly with our lives, sometimes in ways that are nothing short of tragic. Nonetheless, I think it is essential for us to see that psychological problems are ordinary in two very important ways. First, psychological problems are not the product of diseased minds or brains; they arise through the same normal biological and psychological processes as any other aspect of behavior. Second, recent studies have revealed that psychological problems are so much more common in the population than we realized that they cannot be considered to be anything but ordinary.[15]

Psychological Problems Arise in Ordinary Ways
A broad range of variation among individuals in behavior is simply a characteristic of the human race. Human lives are alike in many ways, but individual differences in our behavior are common, natural, and *ordinary*. Individual differences in our behavior arise when ordinary variations in our brains and behavior transact with our experiences. The term *transaction* is discussed in detail in Chapter 9. Briefly, it refers to the processes through which our behavior influences the environments that we experience and, in turn, those experiences influence our behavior. In addition, variations in our individual psychological characteristics influence the extent to which the shocks, frictions, contingencies, and horrors of each person's experiences give rise to psychological problems. These transactional processes lead to adaptive and problematic behavior in exactly the same ways. To repeat myself for emphasis, psychological problems are ordinary in the sense of being caused by the same natural processes as adaptive behavior.[12]

Note that this transactional perspective suggests that some individuals are lucky enough to experience environments that accommodate their individual differences in behavior and do not foster impairing psychological problems, whereas other individuals with similar characteristics transact with unfavorable environments that create distress and dysfunctional behavior. Psychologist Stephen Hinshaw[16] has done a wonderful job of pointing out that psychological problems do not reside in individuals but, rather, in the transactions of individuals with their worlds. Two persons with the same psychological characteristics might differ greatly in their distress and functional impairment if they live in different environments that vary in the extent to which they foster and support adaptive behavior. The adaptiveness of our behavior, therefore, is largely a matter of the *fit* between our behavior and our environments. This is an extremely useful way to think about psychological problems, as it encourages us to think of ways to help others by providing more adaptive environments. It is essential to remember, however, that we each play an active role in creating our own environments.

You may have noticed that Albert Bandura's alternative to the medical model offered a pragmatic definition of *abnormal* behavior. Although his definition was exactly right, we can and definitely should stop referring to our behavior as "abnormal" altogether. Psychological problems are common and arise through ordinary psychological processes; they are not products of an abnormal mind. Thus, my attempt is both to revive Bandura's seminal thinking and to push it further away from judgmental and stigmatizing terms such as abnormal. In addition, it is time to update and expand his views by considering them in the context of important findings from recent research on the nature and prevalence of psychological problems. We have learned a lot in the past 50 years that is directly pertinent to Bandura's views.

Psychological Problems Are Collectively Very Common

The second reason for considering psychological problems to be ordinary phenomena comes from recent data on how common they are. Beginning in the 1990s, large-scale epidemiologic studies[17-19] conducted in the United States and throughout the world have asked tens of thousands of persons in the general population to anonymously answer questions about their feelings, thoughts, perceptions, and actions and the extent to which they are distressing or problematic. These studies have found that people reported panic attacks, episodes of depression, uncontrollable cravings for alcohol, hallucinations, and the entire range of psychological problems at much higher rates than anyone expected. When strict DSM criteria were applied to these reports, approximately 25% of the participants met diagnostic criteria for at least one mental disorder in the past 12 months alone.[20] Each specific mental disorder was not common by itself, but collectively, psychological problems were quite common. We should think critically about these findings, of course, and consider the possibility that the high prevalence of DSM diagnoses of mental disorders revealed in these studies might reflect the overreporting of insignificant problems. Given the stigma against having psychological problems, however, underreporting seems more likely to me. Even under conditions of anonymity, we may not feel comfortable admitting to our fears, obsessions, addictions, distorted perceptions, and the like. Moreover, the psychological problems reported in such studies have been shown not to be trivial but, rather, to be robustly associated with distress and impaired functioning in important areas of people's lives.[21-26] Although some of the psychological problems that people reported in these studies were not the cause of much distress or dysfunction—such as uncomplicated fears of insects or heights—most of the problems identified in these studies were associated with a significant degree of misery and disrupted life functioning.

But, there's much more to be said on this point! As high as the estimate that 25% of adults met DSM criteria for at least one mental disorder in just the past year may seem, it is only the tip of the iceberg! Most of these large studies give us only a snapshot view of human lives during a single year of the lives of the research participants. To fully appreciate how common psychological problems are, however, we need to know the prevalence of psychological problems *across our entire lives*. It is very important, then, that several large studies of the general population have been conducted *longitudinally*, which means that the same persons were asked about their psychological problems multiple times across many years. These longitudinal studies[27] tell us that an eye-popping 80% of people in the general population met DSM diagnostic criteria for at least one mental disorder at least once during the 12–30 years they were studied. Abnormal is starting to look pretty normal!

Furthermore, not all kinds of psychological problems were assessed in these longitudinal studies, so the cumulative proportion of people who meet criteria for at least one from the full list of DSM mental disorders might be even higher if the net had been cast more broadly. Even more important, these studies only reported the prevalence of meeting full DSM diagnostic criteria for a mental disorder. Far more people reported psychological problems that were just below the "official" DSM threshold for a diagnosis. For example, a deeply troubled person who reported feeling sad most of the day nearly every day for at least 2 weeks accompanied by difficulty falling asleep, feelings of worthlessness, and making a concrete plan to commit suicide would exhibit only four "symptoms" of depression and would, therefore, fall below the DSM diagnostic threshold of five symptoms for major depressive disorder and would not qualify for a diagnosis. Thus, the prevalence of depression, to take just one example, was undoubtedly underestimated because the cumulative number of people in these epidemiologic studies who experienced one, two, three, or four distressing and impairing "symptoms" of depression is far greater than the number who exhibited five "symptoms." This is a very important point because there is growing evidence that the numbers of "symptoms" both above and below the DSM diagnostic threshold are associated with misery and interference with our lives in a simple linear way.[10,28]

Many studies have looked closely at persons with "subthreshold" symptoms of mental disorders—people who exhibit some symptoms but not enough to meet DSM diagnostic criteria. To consider a few representative findings, subthreshold post-traumatic stress disorder and subthreshold psychosis are associated with considerable distress and impairment in multiple aspects of life functioning,[29,30] and subthreshold depression in adolescence is associated with the elevated risk for suicide in the future.[31] Therefore, the remarkable finding that most of us will meet full DSM criteria for a mental disorder at some point in our lives understates the ordinariness of psychological problems. When subthreshold numbers of problems are considered, psychological problems are very common, indeed. Indeed, it may be fair to say that nearly all of us will experience psychological problems at some point in our lives.

To reiterate this fundamentally important point, the experience of having psychological problems that are serious enough to be distressing and to interfere with our lives is quite an ordinary thing. Never experiencing a psychological problem is what is not ordinary.[15] If you find these statements to be unreasonable, you may be stigmatizing psychological problems or exaggerating what it means to experience a psychological problem. Although psychological problems can be associated with truly great misery and interference with our lives, some psychological problems make you feel awful for a while, but you get through them okay.[32] Psychological problems can be, but are not always, as serious and different from the usual human experience as we usually think.

Psychological Problems Are Common but Important

Pointing out how ordinary psychological problems are does not mean that we should just endure them. Psychological problems are real and people want help with them. They are important in many ways. From an economic and societal view, the impact of psychological problems on society is huge. The times in our lives when we experience psychological problems are associated with truly massive economic loss due to absenteeism, reduced productivity, and serious impairment in social roles—even more so than any kind of physical health problem.[33–35] Spending more to reduce psychological problems would be a very good financial investment by a society. Sadly, however, far less is spent in essentially all countries to provide help for psychological problems than for physical health problems.[36,37]

This next statement will greatly concern some readers, but it must be said to fully understand the importance of psychological problems: People with serious psychological problems have considerably shorter life expectancies than persons with few such problems.[38,39] For example, attention-deficit/hyperactivity disorder (ADHD), nicotine dependence, and alcohol and opioid misuse directly contribute, respectively, to accidents, cancer, overdoses, and other causes of death.[40–43] In addition, some of the reduced longevity among persons with psychological problems is due to higher rates of suicide in persons with depression and other problems. In other persons with psychological problems, the reduced longevity is caused by poor diets and a failure to obtain necessary medical care.[44] Regardless of the causal pathway, the strong association of psychological problems with reduced longevity underscores the importance of psychological problems. It seems possible to increase longevity by directly helping people with psychological problems, however. For example, large and well-controlled studies found that persons with high levels of ADHD problems (distractibility, impulsivity, etc.) were less likely to attempt suicide[45] and were involved in fewer automobile accidents when they were taking medication for ADHD than when they were not.[46] Successful interventions for other kinds of psychological problems may help as well. Importantly, there also is evidence that it may be possible to offset the health risks due to psychological problems simply by improving physical fitness.[47]

Stigma and Psychological Problems

It is crucially important to recognize that psychological problems can hurt us in two ways. Some variations in our behavior—our moods, fears, or irritability—are inherently distressing. Other psychological problems, such as attention problems, aggression, and social dependence, directly interfere with living a productive and satisfying life. Unfortunately, psychological problems also can hurt us in another way that is totally unnecessary but at least as damaging. Psychological problems are *stigmatized* in nearly all cultures—we look down on people with such problems, we fear them, and we are embarrassed when we have psychological problems ourselves. This stigma makes the lives of people with psychological problems immensely worse.[16,48]

Stigma hurts us in three major ways. First, if we are embarrassed that we feel depressed, for example, that embarrassment can add unnecessary layers of negative feelings that make us even more depressed. Second, stigmatizing our own psychological problems can make it more difficult to seek help when we would benefit from it. Third, the stigma felt by other people about our psychological problems can lead them to treat us as less than fully human, avoid being with us, and create barriers to employment and housing that make our lives far worse. Indeed, stigmatized and uninformed views of psychological problems often lead to unnecessary incarceration and deadly confrontations with police.

Understanding the commonness with which we humans experience psychological problems is one the keys to reducing stigma. Psychological problems are not rarefied things experienced by a few people with diseased minds; they are quite ordinary things experienced by nearly all of us. We have effectively hidden the commonness of psychological problems from ourselves because we so often keep mum about our own problems out of fear of being stigmatized. Hopefully, the findings of recent studies of the high prevalence of psychological problems have opened our eyes. When we understand how ordinary psychological problems are, they lose their frightening and denigrating qualities. When we accept that the great majority of us will experience problems such as fear, anxiety, sadness, or cravings for deadly substances at some time in our lives, it will be more difficult to stigmatize psychological problems.

It is very important to note that we stigmatize psychological problems partly through the words we use, often with the best of intentions. Most of us refer to psychological problems with medical model terms such as *mental illnesses, mental disorders, psychopathology*, or *mental health problems*. We often use these medical model terms in caring ways to imply that the psychological problem is not the person's fault but, rather, is the result of their mental illness. These are profoundly stigmatizing terms, however. Although the denotative meanings of these terms overlap with the definition of psychological problems used in this book, they connote other meanings that are terribly negative and promote stigma. They say that your psychological problems are the result of your *illness, disorder*, and *pathology*. They say that you have psychological problems because your mind is *sick!* How can that not worsen stigma?

It is difficult enough to say about yourself, "I've been unusually unhappy almost all the time for the past month. I just want to sleep all day, I have little appetite, I don't enjoy being with my friends any more, and I feel totally worthless. So, I've decided to get some help because I'm miserable and my work and family life have suffered because of it." But, for most of us, it would be incomparably more difficult to say, "I need professional help because my once healthy mind has become sick—diseased with the mental illness of depression." Thinking about psychological problems as common and ordinary experiences takes away the stigma because it does not imply that the person has an abnormal mind.

Issues that Complicate the Definition of Psychological Problems

Although defining psychological problems pragmatically as behavior that creates levels of distress or impairment that are greater than the risks inherent in seeking help is the only approach that makes sense to me, some very important issues complicate the use of this definition. First, it is well known that some people with psychological problems do not believe they have a problem even when their behavior is viewed as ruining their lives by other well-intentioned people—their families, friends, teachers, and employers. This is frequently the case for persons who exhibit substance abuse, manic behavior, antisocial behavior, and some other problems discussed in Chapters 3–5. In such cases, the decision to provide professional help involves a very complicated and nuanced ethical balancing act. The first effort should always be an attempt to convince such persons that their lives would be better if they received psychological help. In other cases, however, most societies have decided that it is in the best interest of all citizens to enact prevention programs to reduce some kinds of psychological problems, such as chronic antisocial behavior. Furthermore, many governments allow persons to be placed in involuntarily locked psychiatric facilities for several days if they are judged to pose an imminent danger to themselves or others by some combination of mental health professionals, physicians who are not psychiatrists, police officers, and judges. In some cases, the individual can be required to receive treatment involuntarily. Although involuntary confinement and treatment are allowed under laws that were enacted with good intentions, it is a terrifying power that can be and sometimes is abused and must be checked vigilantly.

The second important issue is that the pragmatic definition of psychological problems that I support in this book has cost implications. If people are allowed to decide freely for themselves when they need professional help—and some other persons are pushed into receiving help by others—how much would that cost? Professional help for psychological problems costs money. Currently, psychologists, psychiatrists, other physicians, and others professions are the gatekeepers to such services. In nearly every country, only persons given a reimbursable categorical DSM or ICD diagnosis of a mental disorder can receive services for psychological problems without paying directly for the services. Whether you live in the United States where health insurance companies pay for psychological services—if you are lucky enough to have good health insurance—or live in one of the many countries in which taxpayer-supported services for psychological problems are provided for free, you cannot receive those services without a qualifying diagnosis in virtually every case. Your diagnosis is your only ticket to services, unless you are willing to pay for them yourself.

So, is Bandura's pragmatic definition of psychological problems, which I strongly endorse, naïve? No, it is optimistic, but realistic—in a way that could be *transformative* if it were widely adopted. I can easily imagine societies deciding to provide professional help for psychological problems to all who seek them for one of three reasons. First, it may not increase the number of people who receive services very much. As hard as we fight stigma, many people are reluctant to seek services. And, providers may already be allowing nearly all people seeking professional services to obtain them by providing qualifying diagnoses even when they are not strictly warranted. Thus, the increase in cost may not be great; we will not know until we try.

Second, many societies may decide that providing services to all who believe that they need them would actually save money. As just detailed in this chapter, psychological problems are extremely costly to society in terms of reduced economic productivity and increased physical health problems. There is every reason to believe that increased expenditures for cost-effective methods of preventing and reducing psychological problems would be more than repaid by reductions in the large economic costs of psychological problems to society.[49] People could go back to work, avoid liver problems by not drinking alcohol, reduce their chances of serious injuries because their inattention and impulsivity were under control, and so on.

Third, even if it resulted in increased costs, it would not be unreasonable for a society to decide that spending tax money on reducing psychological problems in everyone who felt the need for help would be one of the most justifiable ways in which public monies could be spent.

Mind–Body Monism

It is important to be crystal clear in my criticisms of the medical model to avoid a misunderstanding. I am definitely not saying that variations in our behavior are not accompanied by variations in our brains. Of course they are; that's just a given. My saying that individual differences in behavior are accompanied by individual differences in the brain does not in any way mean that maladaptive behavior is the result of a *sick* brain, however. Nearly all scientists take a monistic view in which brain and behavior function inseparably—they are just measured at different levels of scientific analysis.[50] Individual differences in behavior that constitute psychological problems are necessarily paralleled by individual differences in the nervous system and vice versa. This is why medications that change the functioning of the nervous system can sometimes help ameliorate psychological problems. Indeed, pharmacologic treatment by physicians is an essential part of helping people with some kinds of psychological problems.[50]

The inseparable parallel of brain and behavior can be seen in other examples. A medical treatment for hepatitis C that is no longer used involved administration of the immune system mediator, interferon-α, which killed the pathogen but also caused marked changes in the brain.[51] These changes in the brain were paralleled by marked and distressing increases in depression, which is one reason why the treatment is now seldom used and has been replaced by one with fewer side effects.

Thus, changes in the brain cause changes in mood; but it works in the opposite direction as well.[52-54] Psychological interventions that reduce psychological problems at the behavioral level also necessarily change the structure and functioning of the brain.[50] Indeed, you could only recall a sentence from this book because reading the book changes your brain! Brain and behavior always change in inseparably parallel ways.

Nonetheless, acknowledging—indeed, emphasizing—the monistic identity of brain and behavior does not in any way justify the stigmatizing medical model of "mental illness" that is used in the DSM. The stigmatizing metaphor of psychological problems as "mental disorders" or "illnesses of the mind" makes the lives of people with psychological problems worse. More than 50 years ago, Bandura[12] put it this way : "Many people who would benefit greatly from psychological treatment avoid seeking help because they fear being stigmatized as mentally deranged" (p. 17).

It should be said that many contemporary psychologists and psychiatrists disagree wholeheartedly with these criticisms of the medical model of psychological problems. Instead, they believe that the medical model provides an effective way of fighting stigma.[55] They think it reduces stigma to think of, for example, a person who is addicted to alcohol or pain killers as suffering from a mental illness or a brain disease. Although I understand and respect their views, I believe we can achieve a far greater reduction in stigma by viewing psychological problems in a very different way: A natural fact of human existence is that we are not all the same. Sometimes our individual differences in behavior are adaptive and sometimes they bite us. Sometimes they create distress and interfere with our lives to the extent that we want help, and hence constitute psychological problems.

There are convincing data that support the view that attributing psychological problems to biological dysfunctions contributes to stigma. Nick Haslam and Erlender Kvalle commented on the published studies of this issue.[56] In the studies they reviewed, for example, descriptions of hypothetical people with various psychological problems were given to mental health professionals. Sometimes the descriptions attributed the psychological problems to a biological dysfunction, such as a deficit in a neurotransmitter in the brain, and sometimes they did not. Across numerous studies, Haslam and Kvalle found that attributing psychological problems to brain dysfunction had mixed blessings in terms of stigma. Although it diminished the extent to which the person was blamed for their problems, it increased stigma by fostering the perception that the person with psychological problems was dangerous, unpredictable, unlikely to get better, and should be avoided. We should avoid stigma, not people with psychological problems.

Admittedly, the term psychological problems as defined in this book is not entirely free of evaluative connotations either—we are talking about "problems" that cause distress and impairment, after all. If we use the term carefully, however, we can avoid the medical model connotations of diseased and deranged minds. Crucially, we do not need to think that we have a sick brain or mind to decide to seek help for a psychological problem. If you play tennis, you do not have to think you have a sick mind to seek help with your serve from a tennis pro. Why not think of seeking help with our emotions or perceptions or behaviors in the same pragmatic and nonstigmatizing way?

Allen Frances and "Saving Normal"

Alan Frances[57] has written a cogent and articulate attack on the DSM-5, called *Saving Normal*. Frances' critique is not entirely novel—it echoes earlier scholarly statements by Stephen Hinshaw[16] and others—but Frances is uniquely qualified to comment on recent editions of the DSM because in addition to being a successful academic psychiatrist, he chaired the task force that developed DSM-IV for the American Psychiatric Association. Note, however, that his criticisms are aimed at DSM-5, not the medical model on which it is based. In my view, Frances' criticism of the DSM is well-intentioned, but with all due respect to a good and decent man, I think his criticism of DSM-5 is exactly backwards.

Frances and I are responding to the same data from recent epidemiologic studies on the commonness of psychological problems that meet DSM diagnostic criteria, but we take opposite messages from it. Frances is disturbed by findings[17-19] that most persons report having experienced psychological problems at some time during their lives. Frances doubts the veracity of this evidence without good grounds, in my opinion. More important, his primary concern is that he believes that each new edition of the DSM has increased the number of persons who meet criteria for a mental disorder diagnosis by including more diagnoses and sometimes relaxing diagnostic criteria.

Frances views this as a problem for three reasons. First, he believes that we should be cautious in labeling people as having a mental disorder because the stigma associated with diagnoses of mental disorder is a major problem. I certainly agree that stigma is a huge problem, but Frances seems to view stigma as inevitable rather than something that can be reduced.

Second, Frances believes there is no defensible definition of mental disorder. Frances[57] states, "'Normal' and mental disorder turn out to be frustratingly elusive—incapable of anything resembling clear, bright-line definition" (p. 33). Frances says this because he is seeking a definition of "mental disorder" in medical model terms, not a simple and pragmatic definition of psychological problems. For Frances, the issue is not the decision to seek help for a psychological problem but, rather, the difference between being "normal" versus having fallen into the abyss of mental illness. Frances[57] asks, "All of us have mild and transient psychiatric symptoms from time to time—does this mean that we are all flirting with mental illness?" (p. 33). His worry is created entirely by imagining there is such a thing as a terrifying abyss of mental illness into which we might slip. Third, he believes that the recent evidence that psychological problems are very common encourages a "medicalizing" of normal human problems and encourages the use of medication for mild problems. This is worrisome to Frances only because he has not given up on the medical model of psychological problems. If we do not view psychological problems as medical conditions that should be treated by physicians, there is no presumption that pharmacological treatments would (or would not) be useful.

Extraordinariness of Psychological Problems

It is important to understand the ways in which psychological problems are ordinary phenomena. Psychological problems are very common and arise in perfectly ordinary ways when individual differences in brain and behavior transact with our experiences. It is equally important, however, to understand that psychological problems can be quite *extraordinary* in two ways. First, psychological problems can feel extraordinarily awful and can impair our lives in deeply destructive ways. Indeed, psychological problems can even lead some people to the extraordinary decision to take their own lives. Second, some psychological problems are quite extraordinary in the sense of being very different from typical behavior. As discussed in later chapters, although most psychological problems involve relatively familiar experiences such as sadness and difficulty paying attention, some psychological problems are characterized by very unusual perceptions and beliefs, by the incomprehensibly sadistic acts of some highly antisocial persons, and by actions that intentionally make one's children physically ill.

We must be very careful how we think about such serious and atypical problems as they challenge our resolve not to think of the persons who experience them as having sick minds. Consider the dimension of psychological problems that result in the diagnosis of schizophrenia, for example. Although most people do not experience any of the problems that define the diagnosis of schizophrenia, there is good evidence from large surveys of the general population for a continuous dimension of these problems, ranging from minor to serious, in the population instead of a binary either–or diagnosis of schizophrenia.[58,59] That is, some people have one schizophrenic problem (e.g., hallucinations) for a brief time, some people chronically experience many of the schizophrenic problems listed in the DSM, and others experience every level of schizophrenic problems between these extremes.[59] Contrary to what the DSM would have us believe, there is not just one group of people who exhibit many symptoms of schizophrenia while the rest of us exhibit none; there is a continuum.

There is also growing evidence that persons with higher levels of schizophrenic problems exhibit differences in brain structure that begin at an early age and become more prominent over time.[58,60] We still have much to learn, but one theory focuses on the normal developmental process in which unneeded neurons in the brain are adaptively pruned from childhood through adolescence. There is a continuum of how rapid and extensive this pruning occurs among people, and it may well be that persons who are more extreme on this continuum are more likely to develop varying degrees of schizophrenic behavior.[61,62] There is no reason why we cannot appropriately think of schizophrenic behavior as a dimension that is paralleled by a dimension of variations in the brain in this way.

Recent research on neuronal pruning and schizophrenic behavior raises an important issue that is very important to address in the context of this book. There is increasing evidence that the higher levels of neuronal pruning during development that are associated with greater schizophrenic behavior are more common in the offspring of women who had infections during pregnancy.[63] The activation of the mother's immune system during pregnancy activates specialized cells in the offspring's brain, called microglia. Microglia are immune cells that protect the brain from infection, but they also destroy unnecessary neurons in the adaptive process of neural pruning. Higher levels of microglial activity due to immune activation could result in higher levels of neural pruning that result in higher levels of schizophrenic behavior.[61,62,64] Thus, this hypothesis suggests that it may be possible to reduce schizophrenic behavior by controlling maternal prenatal infections or by moderating the activity of microglia during synaptic pruning. Such discoveries would be very welcome, of course. They would not challenge the view that psychological problems are best considered to be dimensions of behavior that are paralleled by individual differences in the brain that need not, and should not, be viewed as sick brains. I would never want the dimensional view of psychological problems expressed in this book to discourage biomedical research that might discover individual differences in the brain, endocrine system, or other somatic systems linked to psychological problems that could be moderated with medical treatments. Indeed, such research should be strongly encouraged and accelerated. One does not need to adopt a medical model of psychological problems to do so. One merely needs to accept that mind and body, brain and behavior, are inextricably linked.

References

1. Clark LA, Watson D, Reynolds S. Diagnosis and classification of psychopathology: Challenges to the current system and future directions. *Annual Review of Psychology*. 1995;46:121–153.
2. Kotov R, Krueger RF, Watson D, et al. The Hierarchical Taxonomy of Psychopathology (HiTOP): A dimensional alternative to traditional nosologies. *Journal of Abnormal Psychology*. 2017;126(4):454–477.

3. Krueger RF, Markon KE. A dimensional-spectrum model of psychopathology: Progress and opportunities. *Archives of General Psychiatry.* 2011;68:10–11.

4. Lahey BB, Krueger RF, Rathouz PJ, Waldman ID, Zald DH. A hierarchical causal taxonomy of psychopathology across the life span. *Psychological Bulletin.* 2017;143:142–186.

5. Conway CC, Krueger RF, Board HCE. Rethinking the diagnosis of mental disorders: Data-driven psychological dimensions, not categories, as a framework for mental health research, treatment, and training. *Current Directions in Psychological Science.* In press.

6. Pickworth FA. Agglutination of typhoid and dysentery organisms by the sera of mental hospital patients. *Journal of Pathology and Bacteriology.* 1927;30(4):627–640.

7. Klerman GL. Mental illness, medical model, and psychiatry. *Journal of Medicine and Philosophy.* 1977;2(3):220–243.

8. Freud S. *The standard edition of the complete psychological works of Sigmund Freud.* Oxford, England: Macmillan; 1964.

9. American Psychiatric Association. *Diagnostic and statistical manual of mental disorders.* Fifth ed. Arlington, VA: American Psychiatric Association; 2013.

10. Lahey BB, Applegate B, Barkley RA, et al. DSM-IV field trials for oppositional defiant disorder and conduct disorder in children and adolescents. *American Journal of Psychiatry.* 1994;151:1163–1171.

11. Lahey BB, Applegate B, McBurnett K, et al. DSM-IV field trials for attention-deficit hyperactivity disorder in children and adolescents. *American Journal of Psychiatry.* 1994;151(11):1673–1685.

12. Bandura A. *Principles of behavior modification.* New York, NY: Holt, Rinehart & Winston; 1969.

13. Szasz TS. *Myth of mental illness: Foundations of a theory of personal conduct.* New York, NY: Harper; 1974.

14. Szasz TS. The myth of mental illness. *American Psychologist.* 1960; 15(2):113–118.

15. Moffitt TE, Caspi A, Taylor A, et al. How common are common mental disorders? Evidence that lifetime prevalence rates are doubled by prospective versus retrospective ascertainment. *Psychological Medicine.* 2010;40:899–909.

16. Hinshaw SP. *The mark of shame: Stigma of mental illness and an agenda for change.* New York, NY: Oxford University Press; 2006.

17. Kessler RC, McGonagle KA, Zhao SY, et al. Lifetime and 12-month prevalence of DSM-III-R psychiatric disorders in the United-States—Results from the National Comorbidity Survey. *Archives of General Psychiatry.* 1994;51:8–19.

18. Kessler RC, Aguilar-Gaxiola S, Alonso J, et al. The global burden of mental disorders: An update from the WHO World Mental Health (WMH) surveys. *Epidemiologia e Psichiatria Sociale.* 2009;18(1):23–33.

19. Grant BF, Hasin DS, Stinson FS, et al. Prevalence, correlates, and disability of personality disorders in the United States: Results from the National Epidemiologic Survey on Alcohol and Related Conditions. *Journal of Clinical Psychiatry.* 2004;65(7):948–958.

20. Kessler RC, Chiu WT, Demler O, Walters EE. Prevalence, severity, and comorbidity of 12-month DSM-IV disorders in the National Comorbidity Survey Replication. *Archives of General Psychiatry.* 2005;62(6):617–627.

21. Shaffer D, Fisher P, Dulcan M, et al. The NIMH Diagnostic Interview Schedule for Children (DISC 2.3): Description, acceptability, prevalences, and performance in the MECA study. *Journal of the American Academy of Child and Adolescent Psychiatry.* 1996;35:865–877.

22. Willcutt EG, Nigg JT, Pennington BF, et al. Validity of DSM-IV attention deficit/hyperactivity disorder symptom dimensions and subtypes. *Journal of Abnormal Psychology.* 2012;121:991–1010.

23. Alonso J, Angermeyer MC, Bernert S, et al. Disability and quality of life impact of mental disorders in Europe: Results from the European Study of the Epidemiology of Mental Disorders (ESEMeD) project. *Acta Psychiatrica Scandinavica.* 2004;109:38–46.

24. Kessler RC. The impairments caused by social phobia in the general population: Implications for intervention. *Acta Psychiatrica Scandinavica.* 2003;108:19–27.

25. Kessler RC, Heeringa S, Lakoma MD, et al. Individual and societal effects of mental disorders on earnings in the United States: Results from the National Comorbidity Survey Replication. *American Journal of Psychiatry.* 2008;165:703–711.

26. Copeland WE, Wolke D, Shanahan L, Costello EJ. Adult functional outcomes of common childhood psychiatric problems: A prospective, longitudinal study. *JAMA Psychiatry.* 2015;72(9):892–899.

27. Schaefer JD, Caspi A, Belsky DW, et al. Enduring mental health: Prevalence and prediction. *Journal of Abnormal Psychology.* 2017;126(2):212–224.

28. Lahey BB, Applegate B, McBurnett K, et al. DSM-IV field trials for attention-deficit/hyperactivity disorder in children and adolescents. *American Journal of Psychiatry.* 1994;151:1673–1685.

29. Rosengard RJ, Malla A, Mustafa S, et al. Association of pre-onset subthreshold psychotic symptoms with longitudinal outcomes during treatment of a first episode of psychosis. *JAMA Psychiatry.* 2019;76(1):61–70.

30. Costanzo M, Jovanovic T, Norrholm SD, Ndiongue R, Reinhardt B, Roy MJ. Psychophysiological investigation of combat veterans with subthreshold post-traumatic stress disorder symptoms. *Military Medicine.* 2016;181(8):793–802.

31. Fergusson DM, Horwood LJ, Ridder EM, Beautrais AL. Subthreshold depression in adolescence and mental health outcomes in adulthood. *Archives of General Psychiatry*. 2005;62:66–72.

32. Caspi A, Houts RM, Ambler A, et al. Longitudinal assessment of mental health disorders and comorbidities across 4 decades among participants in the Dunedin Birth Cohort Study. *JAMA Network Open*. 2020;3(4):e203221.

33. Asselmann E, Wittchen HU, Lieb R, Beesdo-Baum K. Sociodemographic, clinical, and functional long-term outcomes in adolescents and young adults with mental disorders. *Acta Psychiatrica Scandinavica*. 2018;137(1):6–17.

34. Kessler RC, Adler L, Ames M, et al. The prevalence and effects of adult attention deficit/hyperactivity disorder on work performance in a nationally representative sample of workers. *Journal of Occupational and Environmental Medicine*. 2005;47(6):565–572.

35. Vigo D, Thornicroft G, Atun R. Estimating the true global burden of mental illness. *Lancet Psychiatry*. 2016;3(2):171–178.

36. Vigo DV, Kestel D, Pendakur K, Thornicroft G, Atun R. Disease burden and government spending on mental, neurological, and substance use disorders, and self-harm: Cross-sectional, ecological study of health system response in the Americas. *Lancet Public Health*. 2019;4(2): E89–E96.

37. Ormel J, Petukhova M, Chatterji S, et al. Disability and treatment of specific mental and physical disorders across the world. *Br J Psychiatry*. 2008;192(5):368–375.

38. Walker ER, McGee RE, Druss BG. Mortality in mental disorders and global disease burden implications: A systematic review and meta-analysis. *JAMA Psychiatry*. 2015;72(4):334–341.

39. Suetani S, Whiteford HA, McGrath JJ. An urgent call to address the deadly consequences of serious mental disorders. *JAMA Psychiatry*. 2015;72(12):1166–1167.

40. Dalsgaard S, Ostergaard SD, Leckman JF, Mortensen PB, Pedersen MG. Mortality in children, adolescents, and adults with attention deficit hyperactivity disorder: A nationwide cohort study. *Lancet*. 2015;385(9983):2190–2196.

41. Poirier AE, Ruan YB, Grevers X, et al. Estimates of the current and future burden of cancer attributable to active and passive tobacco smoking in Canada. *Preventive Medicine*. 2019;122:9–19.

42. Teutsch SM, Naimi TS. Eliminating alcohol-impaired driving fatalities: What can be done? *Annals of Internal Medicine*. 2018;168(8): 587–589.

43. Hser YI, Saxon AJ, Mooney LJ, et al. Escalating opioid dose is associated with mortality: A comparison of patients with and without opioid use disorder. *Journal of Addiction Medicine*. 2019;13(1):41–46.

44. Saha S, Chant D, McGrath J. A systematic review of mortality in schizophrenia—Is the differential mortality gap worsening over time? *Archives of General Psychiatry.* 2007;64(10):1123–1131.

45. Chang Z, Quinn PD, O'Reilly L, et al. Medication for attention-deficit/hyperactivity disorder and risk for suicide attempts. *Biological Psychiatry.* 2020;88(6):452–458.

46. Chang Z, Quinn PD, Hur K, et al. Association between medication use for attention-deficit/hyperactivity disorder and risk of motor vehicle crashes. *JAMA Psychiatry.* 2017;74(6):597–603.

47. Rethorst CD, Leonard D, Barlow CE, Willis BL, Trivedi MH, DeFina LF. Effects of depression, metabolic syndrome, and cardiorespiratory fitness on mortality: Results from the Cooper Center Longitudinal Study. *Psychological Medicine.* 2017;47(14):2414–2420.

48. Hinshaw SP. *Another kind of madness: A journey through the stigma and hope of mental illness.* New York, NY: St. Martin's Press; 2017.

49. Moffitt TE. Psychiatry's opportunity to prevent the rising burden of age-related disease *JAMA Psychiatry.* 2019;76:461–462.

50. Satcher D. Mental health: A report of the surgeon general—Executive summary. *Professional Psychology-Research and Practice.* 2000;31(1):5–13.

51. Dowell NG, Cooper EA, Tibble J, et al. Acute changes in striatal microstructure predict the development of interferon-alpha induced fatigue. *Biological Psychiatry.* 2016;79(4):320–328.

52. Maier SF, Watkins LR. Cytokines for psychologists: Implications of bidirectional immune-to-brain communication for understanding behavior, mood, and cognition. *Psychological Review.* 1998;105(1):83–107.

53. McEwen BS. Brain on stress: How the social environment gets under the skin. *Proceedings of the National Academy of Sciences of the United States of America.* 2012;109:17180–17185.

54. McEwen BS, Bowles NP, Gray JD, et al. Mechanisms of stress in the brain. *Nature Neuroscience.* 2015;18(10):1353–1363.

55. Corrigan PW, Watson AC. At issue: Stop the stigma: Call mental illness a brain disease. *Schizophrenia Bulletin.* 2004;30(3):477–479.

56. Haslam N, Kvaale EP. Biogenetic explanations of mental disorder: The mixed-blessings model. *Current Directions in Psychological Science.* 2015;24(5):399–404.

57. Frances A. *Saving normal: An insider's revolt against out-of-control psychiatric diagnosis, DSM-5, Big Pharma, and the medicalization of ordinary life.* New York, NY: HarperCollins; 2013.

58. Rapoport JL, Giedd JN, Gogtay N. Neurodevelopmental model of schizophrenia: Update 2012. *Molecular Psychiatry.* 2012;17(12):1228–1238.

59. van Os J, Linscott RJ, Myin-Germeys I, Delespaul P, Krabbendam L. A systematic review and meta-analysis of the psychosis continuum: Evidence for a psychosis proneness–persistence–impairment model of psychotic disorder. *Psychological Medicine.* 2009;39(2):179–195.

60. Cannon TD. How schizophrenia develops: Cognitive and brain mechanisms underlying onset of psychosis. *Trends in Cognitive Sciences.* 2015;19(12):744–756.
61. Sellgren CM, Gracias J, Watmuff B, et al. Increased synapse elimination by microglia in schizophrenia patient-derived models of synaptic pruning. *Nature Neuroscience.* 2019;22(3):374–385.
62. Volk DW. Role of microglia disturbances and immune-related marker abnormalities in cortical circuitry dysfunction in schizophrenia. *Neurobiology of Disease.* 2017;99:58–65.
63. Khandaker GM, Zimbron J, Lewis G, Jones PB. Prenatal maternal infection, neurodevelopment and adult schizophrenia: A systematic review of population-based studies. *Psychological Medicine.* 2013;43(2):239–257.
64. Johansson V, Jakobsson J, Fortgang RG, et al. Cerebrospinal fluid microglia and neurodegenerative markers in twins concordant and discordant for psychotic disorders. *European Archives of Psychiatry and Clinical Neuroscience.* 2017;267(5):391–402.

2

From Binary Diagnostic Categories to Dimensions of Psychological Problems

A strong reason was given in Chapter 1 for abandoning the medical model of psychological problems used in the *Diagnostic and Statistical Manual of Mental Disorders* (DSM): The medical model of "mental illness" is based on an analogy that greatly increases stigmatization by unnecessarily attributing psychological problems to terrifying "diseases of the mind." Another strong reason is given in this chapter: The medical model encourages describing different kinds of psychological problems in terms of *binary* (either/or) "diagnoses." According to DSM, there is a clear *discontinuity* between "normal" and "abnormal." That is, a person is either abnormal (i.e., meets criteria for a DSM diagnosis) or normal (i.e., does not meet criteria for a diagnosis). There are no shades of gray in DSM diagnoses, even though there are nothing but shades of gray in reality.

Consider how this kind of binary thinking plays out in practice and why it is a major problem. When a person is ready to push aside the stigma and seek help from a qualified psychologist or other professional, the professional begins by asking questions about the client's life and concerns. This process, which may take a number of sessions, allows the professional to identify the psychological problems for which help is being sought so that options for helping can be discussed. If the services of the professional are covered by the client's health insurance, the helping professional also is gathering enough information to give the person a "diagnosis" of a mental disorder. This does not necessarily mean that the professional adheres to the medical model of psychological problems described in Chapter 1. Whether they do or not, professionals must give the "patient" a diagnosis so the insurance company will pay for the mental health services. Like it or not, this is how the health insurance business works.

Problems of the Binary Diagnostic Approach

Beyond the practical necessity of securing insurance reimbursement, do binary diagnoses help the client and professional choose the best form of help for the client? That is their original purpose, of course. Long before the modern era, proto-physicians such as Hippocrates developed categorical diagnoses of psychological problems. They were trying to place people's problems into the correct binary category so they could generalize what they learned about one person to the next person who came to them for help with the same kind of problems. For example, if the majority of persons classified as "melancholic"—depressed—responded well to a regimen of rest, exercise, and a healthy diet, that would suggest that the next person with melancholia should be offered the same kind of help.

This practice of learning from success makes perfect sense at first blush, but there are a number of important problems inherent in the use of binary diagnoses of psychological problems. First, when we think about psychological problems, we must be careful to think it terms of adjectives and adverbs, not nouns. It is useful for a person to say that they are behaving so *anxiously* in social situations that it may make sense to seek help. We must be careful to avoid speaking of social anxiety in the noun form, however. We run the real and important risk of *reifying* the description of the person's behavior and thinking of social anxiety as a *thing*. Psychological problems are not things, like bacterial infections or broken arms, they refer to individual differences in our emotions, motivations, actions, and thinking that are properly described by adjectives and adverbs. Viewing psychological problems as things fosters rigid dichotomous thinking about them. If social anxiety is a thing, we either have it (we are abnormal) or do not have it (we are normal). In contrast, understanding social anxiety in terms of individual differences allows us to think about the continuum of anxiety in social situations.

Second, it is easy to forget that diagnoses refer to categories of problems, not categories of *people*. It is one thing to say that a person has been behaving in ways that meet diagnostic criteria for schizophrenia, for example, but it is very different to say that the person is "a schizophrenic." That is never appropriate when we think of others or ourselves. The person does not lose their identity as a human being and become a qualitatively different *kind of person* when given a diagnosis of a mental disorder. This is a fundamentally important point because it is much more difficult to swallow the bitter pill of saying "I was a normal person, but now I am a schizophrenic" than saying "I need help because I have started hearing odd voices that no one else hears, and it is distracting me at work and making my friends think I'm weird." Both statements would be difficult for us to make about ourselves, of course, but it is much less stigmatizing to say that you are behaving in a way that you want to change than to say you have become a fundamentally different—sick—kind of person. This less stigmatized way of thinking makes it easier for the person to seek help from a professional who can use what has been learned by science to reduce schizophrenic ways of perceiving, believing, thinking, and relating to others. And, it helps us relate to people who exhibit schizophrenic behavior—or any other kind of psychological problem—in constructive ways.

Diagnoses Are Procrustean Beds

There is another very important reason to avoid binary diagnoses in referring to psychological problems. Diagnostic categories are *Procrustean beds* to an important extent. This means that diagnostic categories distort the specific and unique characteristic of each individual person by implying that everyone who meets criteria for the same diagnosis is exactly—or even mostly—alike. This term comes to us from the Greek myth of the robber baron, Procrustes. Procrustes lived in a house on the well-traveled road between the city of Athens and an important religious site. He offered lodging to wealthy travelers, but while they slept in his iron bed, he acted out his compulsive need to make each traveler fit the bed *exactly* by elongating some parts of their bodies with a hammer and cutting off protruding parts with a sword. Diagnostic categories can act like Procrustean beds in a similar way by encouraging professionals to make the problems of each individual person fit the diagnostic category by stretching some facts and ignoring others.

Ignoring the Extra Bits

In particular, the diagnostic process can create Procrustean beds in which some of the individual's important characteristics are lost. Consider two people who meet DSM diagnostic criteria for generalized anxiety disorder. In this example, both persons have been worried, tense, irritable, restless, and had trouble sleeping for more than 6 months to a degree that is distressing and interferes with their day-to-day lives. Imagine further that one of these persons also experiences enough anxiety during interactions at school and parties that they studiously avoid social situations, whereas the other person is a gregarious socializer who feels that their alcohol and drug use might be getting out of control. Simply considering these two persons to have generalized anxiety disorder would chop off their other issues in a Procrustean manner. That is, focusing only on the diagnosis would ignore each of their individual needs and result in far less than optimal help. I hope this does not happen often in clinical practice, but I strongly suspect that it does.

Polythetic Categories

The DSM defines mental disorders as *polythetic categories*. This means that the diagnosis is based on multiple "symptoms" (i.e., specific psychological problems) that are known to frequently, but not invariably, co-occur. Furthermore, these co-occurring "symptoms" are considered to be equivalent in making diagnoses, which can result in different persons who exhibit different specific psychological problems being given the same diagnosis. I use the DSM diagnosis of "major depressive disorder" to illustrate this point, but the same issue applies to other diagnoses. According to the DSM, there are eight symptoms of major depression. One symptom is intense sadness— also known as dysphoria in DSM-speak. Another is anhedonia— loss of interest or pleasure in things or activities that were formerly valued and enjoyed. According to the DSM, a person may be given the diagnosis of depression if they experience either dysphoria or anhedonia most of the day, nearly every day, for at least 2 weeks. During the time when the person is dysphoric and/or anhedonic, the person also must exhibit a total of at least five "symptoms" of depression, counting dysphoria and anhedonia. The other psychological problems that count toward the diagnosis of major depression include feelings of worthlessness, difficulty concentrating or making decisions, suicidal thoughts or attempts, and changes in so-called vegetative processes—energy, motor movements, sleep, weight, and appetite. In addition, of course, the diagnosis of major depression can only be given if these psychological problems create distress (which is almost guaranteed in the case of depression) and/or impairment in some important area of life functioning, such as school, work, or social relationships.

The polythetic diagnostic criteria for the diagnosis of major depression mean that the diagnosis can be given to people who display very different problematic behaviors, however. One person given this diagnosis may be dysphoric, losing weight unintentionally, feeling worthless, moving in an almost nonstop agitated way, and having great difficulty sleeping and making decisions. In contrast, the same diagnosis of major depression could be given to another person who is not particularly sad but has lost interest in formerly enjoyable things (i.e., is anhedonic) and who moves and speaks slowly, is easily fatigued, sleeps more than usual, has been gaining weight without wanting to, and has been thinking seriously about committing suicide. Note that these two individuals, both of whom meet the diagnostic criteria for major depression, are not alike in *any* of their "symptoms."

Such polythetic diagnostic criteria are based on the assumption that each "symptom" is an indicator of the same underlying problem and that variations in the specific symptoms of each person are relatively unimportant. That is, the assumption is that depression can be manifested in very different ways in different persons. I argue later in this chapter that this is not an entirely unreasonable assumption, but it would be dangerous to accept a strong version of it. Polythetic diagnostic criteria in which each symptom is considered to be the equivalent of every other symptom may be Procrustean beds in the sense of shifting the attention of professionals away from the individual needs of each person. To consider an obvious example, it would be dangerous to consider every person who meets diagnostic criteria for major depression as simply needing to take an antidepressant pill. We should not assume that every pattern of behavior that meets criteria for the same polythetic diagnosis would benefit from the same treatment. At the very least, persons who are actively suicidal would need partly different help than persons who are not.

Diagnoses and the Changeable Nature of Psychological Problems

Binary diagnoses also encourage us to think about psychological problem as fixed and unchanging entities. In the science of botany, there would be great consternation if an apple tree changed into an orange tree a year later. Accurately classified things are supposed to stay in their categorical bins! In contrast, psychological problems sometimes resolve, sometimes persist for a long time, and quite often *change* over time. In one large study of the general population, for example, persons who met diagnostic criteria for major depression were at statistically increased risk for meeting diagnostic criteria 3 years later for *nearly every other DSM diagnosis*.[1] This and other similar studies[2] argue against the increasingly untenable view that "mental disorders" are discrete, fixed, and unchanging entities. As far as psychological problems are concerned, change is not uncommon. This fact is not an anomaly that is unique to the science of psychology, however. Although geologists would be surprised if a block of granite changed into limestone 3 years later, it is well known that mud turns into sedimentary rock and coal turns into diamonds over time under certain conditions. Psychology and psychiatry are only recently taking note of the changes in psychological problems over time and have just begun to study why some changes are more common than others.[1,3,4] This important topic is discussed in greater detail in Chapter 7.

Many DSM Diagnoses of Mental Disorders Are Insufficiently Reliable

The use of binary diagnostic categories is predicated on the assumption that the classification process is *reliable* in clinical practice. This means that a well-trained psychiatrist or psychologist who has the opportunity to interview the same persons seeking help in a clinic twice a few days apart should give the same diagnoses each time. This measure of reliability is referred to as test–retest reliability. To its credit, the Task Force of the American Psychiatric Association that developed the current fifth edition of the DSM conducted a field trial using a number of psychiatric institutions in the United States and Canada to evaluate the test–retest reliability of the most commonly used DSM diagnostic categories. Several hundred clinicians were trained in DSM criteria and then asked to conduct two independent diagnostic assessments of the same persons 1–14 days apart. The Task Force quantified the degree of agreement between the first and second diagnosis using a standard statistical metric of test–retest agreement, called Cohen's kappa, that adjusts for chance agreements.[5] A detailed explanation of Cohen's kappa is provided in the Technical Appendix.

In the DSM-5 field trials, some important kinds of psychological problems were diagnosed with acceptable reliability, including schizophrenia, bipolar disorder, and post-traumatic stress disorder, but a surprising 40% of the DSM-5 diagnoses examined did not reach the conventional cutoff for acceptable reliability, and the diagnosis of alcohol use disorder barely reached the threshold for acceptable test–retest reliability.[6] Of great concern, the test–retest reliability of the diagnoses of major depressive disorder and generalized anxiety disorder were clearly unacceptable. This is disturbing because major depression and generalized anxiety disorder are very common among persons seeking help, and diagnosing these mental disorders is the bread-and-butter of clinical practice. If categorical diagnoses are to be taken seriously, these problems must be diagnosed with high reliability.

There is good and bad news about the often unreliable DSM diagnostic categories: Most professionals do not make diagnoses according to DSM diagnostic criteria![7] This is good news in the sense that it may well be better not to use diagnostic criteria that are not reliable, but it provides cold comfort because diagnoses are often made using idiosyncratic criteria instead. In the real world outside of universities where research is conducted, practitioners often provide diagnoses in an impressionistic way, based on their own understanding of each "mental disorder." This may be especially common among professionals who were not trained in psychiatry, psychiatric social work, or clinical psychology. Why do I mention this fact? It may surprise you, but three-fourths of psychiatric medications are not prescribed by psychiatrists but, rather, by primary care physicians and gynecologists, who are the first to admit they were not adequately trained in the diagnostic criteria.[8,9] For example, when I have given workshops on the psychological problems referred to in the DSM as attention-deficit/hyperactivity disorder (ADHD) to pediatricians, they often tell me that they feel pressured to go beyond their expertise to prescribe medication to every child whose parent says they are not paying attention in school. To justify the prescription to the health insurance provider, they put the diagnosis of ADHD in the child's chart, even when they are not sure if the child's problems actually meet diagnostic criteria for ADHD. This is just my anecdotal experience, of course, and may not reflect pediatric practices in the United States, but I think it does.

Of great concern, there is also reason to believe that unwarranted diagnoses are given in response to fads in society.[10] I once heard a very well-intentioned child psychiatrist speak to a mental health advocacy group about bipolar disorder in children. To my astonishment, he said that bipolar disorder was difficult to recognize because children with bipolar disorder do not exhibit the symptoms of bipolar disorder! Instead, they exhibit symptoms of ADHD and are irritable. This means that he was advocating giving the diagnosis of bipolar disorder to children who met criteria for other well-recognized problems. His book on this topic appears to have played a part in the fourfold increase around the year 2000 in the number of children given the diagnosis of bipolar disorder when they clearly did not meet the DSM criteria for it.[11] In my view, this led to many children being prescribed medications that carry significant risks of side effects with questionable justification.

Dimensions of Psychological Problems Instead of Binary Diagnoses

What is the alternative to binary diagnoses of mental disorders? How should we think about and study psychological problems? Many psychologists and psychiatrists now advocate describing psychological problems in *dimensional* instead of categorical terms.[12,13] What does this mean?

Extensive research tells us that some specific psychological problems are correlated with one another more than they are correlated with other problems. This means that some sets of psychological problems tend to co-occur often—if you have one, you are more likely than chance to have one or more of the others. For example, the specific psychological problems that are considered to be "symptoms" of major depression are more correlated with one another than they are with the "symptoms" that define, for example, ADHD. If you are deeply sad, you are also likely to experience sleep problems and have the other problems that define major depression. Such correlations are not perfect, but they are pretty substantial.

Therefore, instead of defining major depression as a categorical diagnosis that is present if all of the required "symptoms" are experienced and absent when they are not, we can simply define depression as a *dimension* based on the number and severity of the correlated psychological problems that the person experiences. For example, if we count problems (ignoring their severity for the sake of simplicity), Person 1 might exhibit three depressive problems (e.g., anhedonia, lethargy, and feelings of worthless), another person may exhibit four problems (e.g., dysphoria, problems sleeping, loss of appetite, and suicidal thoughts), a third person might experience zero depression problems, and so on. We can quantify a dimension of depression on which everyone has a score, from zero to the highest number. And we can do the same thing for the other correlated sets of psychological problems.

Some people will have high levels of one kind of correlated problems, others may be high on more than one dimension, and others will have one or two problems from each of several different dimensions. That heterogeneity among people and their problems tends to get ignored when we focus on categorical diagnoses, but it is easily captured and quantified in dimensional approaches.

Why is a dimensional approach to psychological problems better than the DSM approach based on categorical diagnoses? Let me count the ways (pun intended):

1. Dimensional approaches are not based on the terrifying assumption that persons who meet diagnostic criteria for a mental disorder are "mentally ill." In a binary diagnostic approach, everyone in the population is considered to be "normal," except for persons who meet diagnostic criteria for a mental disorder, who are considered to be "abnormal." Using the categorical diagnostic approach, a person who reports four "symptoms" of major depression is perfectly normal but is just one "symptom" away from falling into the abyss of "mental illness." This unsettling view is nonsensical in a dimensional approach. Everyone is somewhere on the natural continuum of depression—from not all to very much—and each person can choose to seek help at any point on the continuum that makes sense.

2. Binary diagnoses may discourage help for persons with problems that are just below the threshold of the diagnostic criteria. In a dimensional approach, it makes good sense for a person who is dysphoric, anhedonic, easily fatigued, and feeling worthless to decide to seek help even though they do not quite meet DSM criteria for major depression. Indeed, as discussed in Chapter 1, persons with "subthreshold" psychological problems very often want and can benefit from help. To be fair to the DSM-5, it has begun to move toward the dimensional perspective advocated in this book. The introduction to DSM-5 states, "Clinicians may thus encounter individuals whose symptoms do not meet full criteria for a mental disorder but who demonstrate a clear need of treatment or care" (p. 20).[14] Therefore, in clinical practice, diagnoses of mental disorders are sometimes intentionally given to people who do not meet criteria for any diagnosis. If a person whose spouse asked for a divorce 2 years ago is still feeling deeply sad, hopeless about the future, and is having trouble sleeping, a professional might provide treatment for major depression even

though the person only exhibits three "symptoms" instead of the five required by the DSM. That is reasonable for that person, of course, but if a system of categorical diagnoses only works if it has fuzzy lower boundaries, it makes more sense to me to move to a fully dimensional approach.

3. Dimensional ratings of psychological problems are far more reliable than categorical diagnoses.[15–17] This is partly due to the statistical advantages of continuous versus binary measurements of all kinds, but it is a commonsense issue as well. In a test–retest study, if a person changes one aspect of what they reported in the first interview (e.g., saying that they felt sad nearly every day in the first interview but reporting feeling sad on just half of the days in the past 2 weeks in the second interview), the whole diagnosis would change from "present" to "absent." In a dimensional approach to depression, that small change would result in only a small difference in the continuous depression rating. Psychological problems are not difficult to measure reliably; they only appear to be when we impose unjustifiable binary categories on them.

4. Dimensional ratings of psychological problems are more valid than categorical diagnoses.[17] What does this mean? One important way to evaluate the validity of a measure of psychological problems is to see if it is associated with other important things to which it should be related. For example, if the diagnosis of ADHD is valid, children given the diagnosis of ADHD should perform less well on average in the classroom than children who exhibit few of these problems. This correlation between the binary diagnosis and impaired functioning provides evidence for the validity of the diagnosis. Crucially, when both binary and dimensional measures of psychological problems are tested for validity in this way, the validity correlations are considerably stronger for dimensional than categorical measures.[17] In the example of ADHD again, this is probably because the categorical diagnosis misses the substantial number of persons with "subthreshold" levels of ADHD problems (i.e., just below the threshold for the diagnosis) who are impaired in the classroom and at work.[18,19]

5. Dimensional approaches do not require *differential diagnosis*. Professionals who use the DSM diagnostic approach often have to make the difficult decision that the individual should be viewed as meeting one diagnosis versus another diagnosis. The difficulty is that the diagnosis that is chosen often does not reflect the fact that problems of both kinds are present and the differential diagnosis could easily have gone the other way. In contrast, the dimensional approach encourages helping professionals to rate every dimension of psychological problems to gain a comprehensive assessment of all of the psychological problems experienced by the person seeking help. To be fair, one can give multiple "comorbid" diagnoses using the categorical approach, but this is discouraged and even restricted by rules in the DSM that do not allow many pairs of diagnoses to both be given. For example, persons who meet diagnostic criteria for both generalized anxiety disorder and major depression can only be given the diagnosis of major depression. This Procrustean rule simply lops off the worry and tension by artificially prioritizing the diagnosis of depression.

Child and adolescent psychologists and psychiatrists have used dimensional measures for many years.[20,21] Thus, many of them are already quite comfortable with dimensional assessments of psychological problems. Much less work has been done to develop dimensional measures of psychological problems for adults, however. Thus, I am advocating a jolting revolution for most psychologists and psychiatrists who work with adults. Moving from categorical to dimensional assessments of psychological problems will feel like a major paradigm shift for clinicians who have solely focused on adult psychological problems from a DSM diagnostic perspective. The thesis of this book is that it is a necessary revolution that will be well worth the effort.

Dichotomous Decisions to Treat or Not Treat

Even when one conceptualizes psychological problems in terms of individual differences that lie on continua rather than as categorical disease entities, it is necessary for the person to decide when to seek help. That means that the person and the professional need to make the *inherently binary decision to treat or not treat*.[22] Therefore, the natural continuum of, for example, generalized must be dichotomized in this practical sense when the level of worry is bothersome enough to seek help. As explicitly noted in Chapter 1, this decision is up to the individual seeking help, but hopefully in consultation with the professional and others.

Therefore, to allow helping professionals to constructively assist in this decision, it is important to use research to give helping professionals as much empirical guidance as possible on the optimal point on each continuum of psychological problems to make the decision to treat.

The necessity of dichotomizing dimensions of psychological problems to make this pragmatic binary decision is why many psychologists and psychiatrists, myself included, have spent years of their careers conducting research to help identify the points of inflection on each dimension of psychological problems above which the degree of distress and functional impairment may be too substantial to ignore. I say "may be too substantial to ignore" because this kind of research can only tell us how much functional impairment is associated with each number of problems in the population *on average*, and each individual is different. The threshold that is appropriate for one person may differ from what is appropriate on average. Everyone is different, and conventional thresholds will not apply to every unique individual. This issue is avoided in the dimensional approach advocated in this book. Help can be sought when each individual thinks it makes sense anywhere on the continuum of psychological problems.

Describing the Dimensions of Psychological Problems

What are the dimensions of psychological problems that should replace binary diagnoses? In the next three chapters, I describe the major dimensions of psychological problems at multiple levels using the following terms:

1. *Specific problems*: When I refer to *specific* psychological problems in this chapter, I am usually describing in a granular way problems that are treated as "symptoms" in the medical-model

language of the DSM. Examples are difficulty falling asleep, frequently losing one's temper, or needing to check that all of the doors and windows in the house are locked exactly seven times before going to bed.

2. *Dimensions of problems*: Dimensions are sets of multiple specific psychological problems that are highly correlated with one another, to the extent that they can be summed to define dimensions. In the following chapters, I will often be able to describe the dimensions of psychological problems based on strong empirical evidence, but there are some unfortunate gaps in that evidence. As psychology and psychiatry have increasingly moved toward dimensional views of psychological problems, it has become clear that not all correlations among all specific psychological problems ever have been calculated! We have exhaustively studied the correlations among many psychological problems, especially in children and adolescents,[16,20,23,24] but much remains to be learned about other sets of problems. Therefore, Chapters 3–5 properly should be viewed as one psychologist's best guesses—hypotheses— regarding the dimensions of psychological problems based on the currently existing evidence. To make this concept of dimensions of psychological problems more concrete, consider the dimension of "attention problems." The dimension of attention problems is defined by the number and severity of specific problems in maintaining selective attention and staying organized as we attempt to execute tasks. Many studies make it clear that nine problems in maintaining attention are so highly correlated with one another that they can be considered to define the dimension of attention problems.[18] In the dimensional approach to psychological problems advocated in this book, this means that a continuous dimensional scale of attention problems can be created by having people rate the frequency and severity of each of these specific problems, such as on a scale of 0 = not at all, 1 = just a little, 2 = pretty much, and 3 = very much. Because we know a great deal from studies about these nine specific attention problems, defining the dimension of attention problems is straightforward and well supported by evidence. In technical terms, these nine problems co-occur so often

that the statistical method of factor analysis indicates they define a coherent "first-order" dimension of psychological problems.[18] Factor analysis is discussed further in the Technical Appendix. Note that such dimensions are polythetic, like diagnostic categories, which means that each problem is considered to be equivalent to each other problem in defining the continuous dimension of attention problems. I think that is justified, but we have to be very careful to remember that every person with the same quantitative score on the dimension of attention problems does not exhibit the same specific problems.

3. *Second-order dimensions*: I have organized Chapters 3–5 around the three *second-order factors* listed at the top of Figure 2.1: internalizing, externalizing, and problems of thought and affect. Second-order dimensions are defined by patterns of *correlations among dimensions*. For example, the dimensions reflecting fears, worries, and depression are correlated with one another more than they are correlated with other dimensions. This means that if persons experience some of the problems in the worries dimension, their likelihood of experiencing other problems in the fears and depression dimensions is higher than average. Similarly, the second-order dimensions of ADHD,

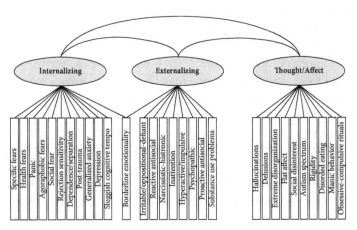

Figure 2.1 Hypothesized second-order internalizing, externalizing, and psychotic thought/affect dimensions of psychological problems.

antisocial behavior, and substance use problems also are highly correlated with one another.[25-27] By tradition, the first group of correlated problems have long been referred to as *internalizing problems*, whereas the latter are known as *externalizing problems*.[28,29] These outdated terms harken back to Freudian notions of "acting out"— externalizing—mental conflicts versus internalizing such conflicts. Few psychologists and psychiatrists still endorse Freudian views, but we are stuck with the terms. They are used in the names of the next two chapters, so it is important to remember that I am using them only descriptively. Although much more remains to be learned, correlations among dimensions reflecting psychotic cognition, social disinterest, and related problems appear to define the second-order dimension of thought and affect problems.

To reiterate a key point, the second-order dimensions of psychological problems defined in Chapters 3–5, and the correlations among them that are illustrated in Figure 2.1, are based on educated guesses. These guesses are based on a growing number of informative studies[16,23,25,27,30-54] that provide relevant empirical information, but much remains to be learned. I feel reasonably confident in organizing the three following chapters in this hierarchical way, but there are important gaps in our knowledge that require some guesswork.

In particular, some very important dimensions have almost never been included in our studies of the correlational structure of dimensions of problems. This is not because these are newly recognized psychological problems—they have been described for more than 100 years—but because psychologists and psychiatrists have only recently changed how they study them. These dimensions of problems, which were formerly conceptualized as "personality disorders," have often been largely ignored by most researchers in psychiatry and psychology because they were thought to be fundamentally different from the other mental disorders. They were thought to be untreatable problems resulting from malformed personalities rather than "mental illnesses" that result from "breakdowns" of normal personalities. This distinction was completely unfounded[55,56] and left us with incomplete information about many serious psychological problems.

Therefore, I have had to make less well-substantiated guesses based on the limited amount of empirical evidence available in placing these erstwhile personality disorder dimensions in the organizational structure of this chapter illustrated in Figure 2.1. Any time one attempts to pause to take stock of what has been learned in a field, gaps in current knowledge will make some statements uncomfortably tentative. As many psychologists and psychiatrists are saying as loudly as they can,[13,15,57,58] a great deal more research is needed to put our descriptions of the nature of psychological problems on a truly firm empirical foundation. The encouraging news is that the recent 11th edition of the *International Classification of Diseases*, published by the World Health Organization, has replaced the categorical diagnoses of personality disorders with dimensions.[59] Although much remains to be learned about these dimensions of psychological problems, I believe this is a move in the right direction.

Foreshadowing what will be detailed in later chapters, it will help you to know that a central tenet of this book is that psychological problems are correlated enough to define dimensions because they are partly influenced by the same genetic and environmental causal risk factors and partly share the same brain mechanisms. As you read about the highly correlated dimensions that define second-order dimensions of psychological problems, keep in mind that these dimensions are similarly hypothesized to be correlated because they share causes and mechanisms at this higher level.[13] Furthermore, it is important to note that the curved lines that connect the second-order dimensions of psychological problems in Figure 2.1 mean that even the second-order dimensions are substantially correlated with one another. You may be surprised to learn this, but every specific psychological problem, every dimension of problems, and even every second-order dimension of psychological problems is positively correlated with the others. This means that it is common for problems from different dimensions to co-occur in the same persons. As addressed in Chapter 6, these important correlations are hypothesized to reflect some highly nonspecific causes and mechanisms that underlie *every* dimension of psychological problems.[13]

Let me make the fundamentally important point that all dimensions of psychological problems are correlated with one another in a different way. Figure 2.1 should not be interpreted as depicting *separate silos* containing different groups of psychological problems. All psychological problems are positively correlated to varying degrees. People generally do not experience the "symptoms" of a single DSM-5 "mental disorder"; rather, they experience a *mishmash* of psychological problems. Some specific problems are frequently experienced together; they are the highly correlated sets of problems that define each dimension. Nonetheless, because every dimension is positively correlated with every other dimension to some degree, we are more likely than chance to experience problems from other dimensions. Almost no one experiences, for example, six inattention problems and no other problems. Instead, we mostly experience *admixtures* of problems from multiple dimensions. These admixtures of problems from correlated dimensions are to be expected in the dimensional approach. In contrast, admixtures of psychological problems are viewed as troubling violations of the sharp boundaries that should divide supposedly distinct categorical diagnoses in the DSM. That is one of the primary shortcomings of the binary diagnostic approach and a sufficient reason by itself for leaving it behind. Mother nature is messy and does not respect binary diagnostic categories. In nature, psychological problems are dimensional, correlated, and mishmashed. One advantage of the dimensional approach is that it encourages us to rate every dimension of psychological problems to comprehensively evaluate the needs of the person.

Cross-Cutting Issues

Before describing the various dimensions of psychological problems in detail, however, I need to make three more important general points. First, you will notice as you read Chapters 3–5 that some specific psychological problems are part of *multiple* dimensions. Irritability, anhedonia (reduced pleasure), difficulty concentrating, variations in levels of motor activity, changes in sleep patterns, and talkativeness are examples of problems that are part of several different dimensions.[27] Much remains to be learned about these problems, but it is possible that they reveal something important about what multiple dimension of psychological problems share in common.

Second, let me preview the complex issue of problems in social relationships. By definition, our behavior only constitutes a psychological problem if it causes us distress or interferes with our lives. And, given that we humans are social animals, interference with our social relationships is an important part of the impairment that defines a psychological problem. As you read Chapters 3–5, you will see that there are many *quite different* ways of behaving that interfere with initiating and maintaining meaningful relationships with other persons. These include diminished interest in having relationships with others in the first place; insecurity and sensitivity to rejection by others to an extent that interferes with relationships; distrusting and suspecting others of infidelity and malicious intent without cause; an entitled need for others to treat us as being special and superior; alienating others by being clinging, dependent, demanding, selfish, and emotionally manipulative; driving away others by being violent, criminal, or by abusing alcohol or drugs; upsetting others by moralistically holding them to unreasonably high and inflexible moral standards; excessive involvement in work that detracts from our relationships; alienating others by having ideas, perceptions, or behaviors that seem disturbingly distorted to them; and deficits in the basic skills of reciprocal social interaction, such as respecting the personal physical boundaries of others. Thus, difficulty in social relationships is an outcome of many different kinds of psychological problems. You will see the many different patterns of behavior that interfere with adaptive social relationships in the descriptions of dimensions of psychological problems in Chapters 3–5.

Finally, when I describe the multiple specific psychological problems that are correlated enough to define each dimension, be careful not to misinterpret these lists as meaning that a person must exhibit all of the listed problems to be said to be troubled by that dimension of behavior. A person can experience any number of those problems. We are speaking about *continuous* dimensions on which a person may have anything from no problems to extreme problems. The extent to which each person can be said to experience each dimension of psychopathology to different extents will reflect both the number of specific problems they experience and the severity of the problems that cause them distress and impair functioning in their lives.

References

1. Lahey BB, Zald DH, Hakes JK, Krueger RF, Rathouz PJ. Patterns of heterotypic continuity associated with the cross-sectional correlational structure of prevalent mental disorders in adults. *JAMA Psychiatry.* 2014;71:989–996.

2. Asselmann E, Wittchen HU, Lieb R, Beesdo-Baum K. Sociodemographic, clinical, and functional long-term outcomes in adolescents and young adults with mental disorders. *Acta Psychiatrica Scandinavica.* 2018;137(1):6–17.

3. Plana-Ripoll O, Pedersen CB, Holtz Y, et al. Exploring comorbidity within mental disorders among a Danish national population. *JAMA Psychiatry.* 2019;76(3):259–270.

4. Caspi A, Houts RM, Ambler A, et al. Longitudinal assessment of mental health disorders and comorbidities across 4 decades among participants in the Dunedin Birth Cohort Study. *JAMA Network Open.* 2020;3(4):e203221.

5. Cohen J. A coefficient of agreement for nominal scales. *Educational and Psychological Measurement.* 1960;20(1):37–46.

6. Regier DA, Narrow WE, Clarke DE, et al. DSM-5 field trials in the United States and Canada, Part II: Test–retest reliability of selected categorical diagnoses. *American Journal of Psychiatry.* 2013;170:59–70.

7. First MB, Bhat V, Adler D, et al. How do clinicians actually use the *Diagnostic and Statistical Manual of Mental Disorders* in clinical practice and why we need to know more. *Journal of Nervous and Mental Disease.* 2014;202(12):841–844.

8. Karanges EA, Stephenson CP, McGregor IS. Longitudinal trends in the dispensing of psychotropic medications in Australia from 2009–2012: Focus on children, adolescents and prescriber specialty. *Australian and New Zealand Journal of Psychiatry.* 2014;48(10):917–931.

9. Mark TL, Levit KR, Buck JA. Psychotropic drug prescriptions by medical specialty. *Psychiatric Services.* 2009;60(9):1167.

10. Hinshaw SP, Scheffler RM. *The ADHD explosion: Myths, medication, money, and today's push for performance.* New York, NY: Oxford University Press; 2014.

11. Blader JC, Carlson GA. Increased rates of bipolar disorder diagnoses among US child, adolescent, and adult inpatients, 1996–2004. *Biological Psychiatry.* 2007;62(2):107–114.

12. Krueger RF, Kotov R, Watson D, et al. Progress in achieving quantitative classification of psychopathology. *World Psychiatry.* 2018;17(3):282–293.

13. Lahey BB, Krueger RF, Rathouz PJ, Waldman ID, Zald DH. A hierarchical causal taxonomy of psychopathology across the life span. *Psychological Bulletin.* 2017;143:142–186.

14. American Psychiatric Association. *Diagnostic and statistical manual of mental disorders.* Fifth ed. Arlington, VA: American Psychiatric Association; 2013.

15. Helzer JE, Kraemer HC, Krueger RF. The feasibility and need for dimensional psychiatric diagnoses. *Psychological Medicine.* 2006;36(12):1671–1680.

16. Lahey BB, Rathouz PJ, Applegate B, et al. Testing structural models of DSM-IV symptoms of common forms of child and adolescent psychopathology. *Journal of Abnormal Child Psychology.* 2008;36:187–206.

17. Markon KE, Chmielewski M, Miller CJ. The reliability and validity of discrete and continuous measures of psychopathology: A quantitative review. *Psychological Bulletin.* 2011;137:856–879.

18. Willcutt EG, Nigg JT, Pennington BF, et al. Validity of DSM-IV attention deficit/hyperactivity disorder symptom dimensions and subtypes. *Journal of Abnormal Psychology.* 2012;121:991–1010.

19. Lahey BB, Applegate B, McBurnett K, et al. DSM-IV field trials for attention-deficit hyperactivity disorder in children and adolescents. *American Journal of Psychiatry.* 1994;151(11):1673–1685.

20. Achenbach TM, Conners CK, Quay HC, Verhulst FC, Howell CT. Replication of empirically derived syndromes as a basis for taxonomy of child and adolescent psychopathology. *Journal of Abnormal Child Psychology.* 1989;17:299–323.

21. Quay HC. Classification. In: Quay HC, Werry JS, eds. *Psychopathological disorders of childhood.* 3rd ed. New York, NY: Wiley; 1986:1–42.

22. Widiger TA. Considering the research: Commentary on "The trait-type dialectic: Construct validity, clinical utility, and the diagnostic process." *Personality Disorders: Theory Research and Treatment.* 2019;10(3):215–219.

23. Lahey BB, Applegate B, Waldman ID, Loft JD, Hankin BL, Rick J. The structure of child and adolescent psychopathology: Generating new hypotheses. *Journal of Abnormal Psychology.* 2004;113:358–385.

24. Forbes MK, Sunderland M, Rapee RM, et al. A detailed hierarchical model of psychopathology: From individual symptoms up to the general factor of psychopathology. *Clinical Psychological Science.* 2021;9:139–168.

25. Ivanova MY, Achenbach TM, Rescorla LA, et al. Syndromes of self-reported psychopathology for ages 18–59 in 29 societies. *Journal of Psychopathology and Behavioral Assessment.* 2015;37(2):171–183.

26. Krueger RF, Markon KE, Patrick CJ, Iacono WG. Externalizing psychopathology in adulthood: A dimensional-spectrum conceptualization and its implications for DSM-V. *Journal of Abnormal Psychology.* 2005;114:537–550.

27. Lahey BB, Zald DH, Perkins SF, et al. Measuring the hierarchical general factor model of psychopathology in young adults. *International Journal of Methods in Psychiatric Research.* 2018;27:e1593.

28. Achenbach TM. Classification of children's psychiatric symptoms: A factor analytic study. *Psychological Monographs.* 1966;80:1–37.
29. Krueger RF, Caspi A, Moffitt TE, Silva PA. The structure and stability of common mental disorders (DSM-III-R): A longitudinal–epidemiological study. *Journal of Abnormal Psychology.* 1998;107:216–227.
30. Bedford A, Deary IJ. The British Inventory of Mental Pathology (BIMP): Six factored scales. *Personality and Individual Differences.* 2006;40(5):1017–1025.
31. Becker DF, McGlashan TH, Grilo CM. Exploratory factor analysis of borderline personality disorder criteria in hospitalized adolescents. *Comprehensive Psychiatry.* 2006;47(2):99–105.
32. Burt SA. Do etiological influences on aggression overlap with those on rule breaking? A meta-analysis. *Psychological Medicine.* 2013;43:1801–1812.
33. Forbes MK, Kotov R, Ruggero CJ, Watson D, Zimmerman M, Krueger RF. Delineating the joint hierarchical structure of clinical and personality disorders in an outpatient psychiatric sample. *Comprehensive Psychiatry.* 2017;79:19–30.
34. Fossati A, Beauchaine TP, Grazioli F, Carretta I, Cortinovis F, Maffei C. A latent structure analysis of *Diagnostic and Statistical Manual of Mental Disorders,* fourth edition, narcissistic personality disorder criteria. *Comprehensive Psychiatry.* 2005;46(5):361–367.
35. Kotov R, Ruggero CJ, Krueger RF, Watson D, Yuan QL, Zimmerman M. New dimensions in the quantitative classification of mental illness. *Archives of General Psychiatry.* 2011;68(10):1003–1011.
36. Krueger RF, Markon KE, Patrick CJ, Iacono WG. Externalizing psychopathology in adulthood: A dimensional-spectrum conceptualization and its implications for DSM-V. *Journal of Abnormal Psychology.* 2005;114(4):537–550.
37. Lewis K, Caputi P, Grenyer BFS. Borderline personality disorder subtypes: A factor analysis of the DSM-IV criteria. *Personality and Mental Health.* 2012;6(3):196–206.
38. Markon KE. Modeling psychopathology structure: A symptom-level analysis of Axis I and II disorders. *Psychological Medicine.* 2010;40:273–288.
39. Waszczuk MA, Kotov R, Ruggero C, Gamez W, Watson D. Hierarchical structure of emotional disorders: From individual symptoms to the spectrum. *Journal of Abnormal Psychology.* 2017;126(5):613–634.
40. den Hollander-Gijsman ME, Wardenaar KJ, de Beurs E, et al. Distinguishing symptom dimensions of depression and anxiety: An integrative approach. *Journal of Affective Disorders.* 2012;136(3):693–701.
41. Boudreaux MJ, South SC, Oltmanns TF. Symptom-level analysis of DSM-IV/DSM-5 personality pathology in later life: Hierarchical structure and predictive validity across self- and informant ratings. *Journal of Abnormal Psychology.* 2019;128(5):365–384.

42. Sanislow CA, Grilo CM, McGlashan TH. Factor analysis of the DSM-III-R borderline personality disorder criteria in psychiatric inpatients. *American Journal of Psychiatry.* 2000;157(10):1629-1633.
43. Yen S, Shea MT, Sanislow CA, et al. Borderline personality disorder criteria associated with prospectively observed suicidal behavior. *American Journal of Psychiatry.* 2004;161(7):1296-1298.
44. Lahey BB, Applegate B, Hakes JK, Zald DH, Hariri AR, Rathouz PJ. Is there a general factor of prevalent psychopathology during adulthood? *Journal of Abnormal Psychology.* 2012;121(4):971-977.
45. Warren JI, Burnette M. Factor invariance of Cluster B psychopathology among male and female inmates and association with impulsive and violent behavior. *Journal of Forensic Psychiatry & Psychology.* 2012;23(1):40-60.
46. Constantino JN, Davis SA, Todd RD, et al. Validation of a brief quantitative measure of autistic traits: Comparison of the Social Responsiveness Scale with the Autism Diagnostic Interview–Revised. *Journal of Autism and Developmental Disorders.* 2003;33(4):427-433.
47. Blevins CA, Weathers FW, Witte TK. Dissociation and posttraumatic stress disorder: A latent profile analysis. *Journal of Traumatic Stress.* 2014;27(4):388-396.
48. Michelini G, Barch DM, Tian Y, Watson D, Klein DN, Kotov R. Delineating and validating higher-order dimensions of psychopathology in the Adolescent Brain Cognitive Development (ABCD) study. *Translational Psychiatry.* 2019;9(1):261-396.
49. Blanco C, Krueger RF, Hasin DS, et al. Mapping common psychiatric disorders: structure and predictive validity in the National Epidemiologic Survey on Alcohol and Related Conditions. *JAMA Psychiatry.* 2013;70(2):199-208.
50. Blanco C, Wall MM, He JP, et al. The space of common psychiatric disorders in adolescents: Comorbidity structure and individual latent liabilities. *Journal of the American Academy of Child and Adolescent Psychiatry.* 2015;54(1):45-52.
51. Forbush KT, Watson D. The structure of common and uncommon mental disorders. *Psychological Medicine.* 2013;43(1):97-108.
52. Foss-Feig JH, Velthorst E, Smith L, et al. Clinical profiles and conversion rates among young individuals with autism spectrum disorder who present to clinical high risk for psychosis services. *Journal of the American Academy of Child and Adolescent Psychiatry.* 2019;58(6):582-588.
53. Addington J, Cornblatt BA, Cadenhead KS, et al. At clinical high risk for psychosis: outcome for nonconverters. *American Journal of Psychiatry.* 2011;168(8):800-805.
54. Petersen SM, Toftdahl NG, Nordentoft M, Hjorthoj C. Schizophrenia is associated with increased risk of subsequent substance abuse

diagnosis: A nation-wide population-based register study. *Addiction.* 2019;114(12):2217–2226.

55. Frances AJ, First MB, Widiger TA, et al. An A to Z guide to DSM-IV conundrums. *Journal of Abnormal Psychology.* 1991;100(3):407–412.
56. Clark LA, Watson D, Reynolds S. Diagnosis and classification of psychopathology: Challenges to the current system and future directions. *Annual Review of Psychology.* 1995;46:121–153.
57. Eaton NR, Krueger RF, Keyes KM, et al. Borderline personality disorder co-morbidity: Relationship to the internalizing–externalizing structure of common mental disorders. *Psychological Medicine.* 2011;41:1041–1050.
58. Kotov R, Krueger RF, Watson D, et al. The Hierarchical Taxonomy of Psychopathology (HiTOP): A dimensional alternative to traditional nosologies. *Journal of Abnormal Psychology.* 2017;126(4):454–477.
59. Oltmanns JR. Personality traits in the *International Classification of Diseases* 11th revision (ICD-11). *Current Opinion in Psychiatry.* 2021;34(1):48–53.

3

Dimensions of Internalizing Problems

Until now, I have discussed the best way to think about psychological problems using only a few examples of dimensions of psychological problems to illustrate my points. In this and the following two chapters, I describe the major dimensions of psychological problems that complicate, disturb, and partly define human lives. A few points need to be made before beginning the description of these dimensions of psychological problems, however. First, although Chapters 3–5 cover many dimensions of psychological problems, it is not entirely comprehensive. To keep the message of this book manageable in scope, I am not mentioning every one of the many psychological problems that we humans experience. Second, although psychologists have been studying the dimensions of psychological problems for decades, there is still much we do not know, particularly about the dimensions of psychological problems in adults. This means that I can sometimes use solid data to describe dimensions of psychological problems, but at other times I present tentative hypotheses that must be tested. Third, although a number of diagnoses of *Diagnostic and Statistical Manual of Mental Disorders* (DSM) mental disorders can be thought of as dichotomized versions of some of the continuous dimensions presented in Chapters 3–5, that is not always the case. Some DSM diagnostic categories do not align well with dimensions of psychological problems. For example, as detailed later in this chapter, the diagnosis of post-traumatic stress disorder (PTSD) is a DSM diagnostic category that seems to be defined by more than one dimension of psychological problems. I am raising the very real possibility that some DSM diagnostic categories reflect heterogeneous admixtures of more than one dimension of psychological problems. This proposition can only be evaluated when research has been conducted on broader sets of psychological problems than has been conducted to date, so it is just scientific food for thought at this point.

In this chapter, I describe a number of dimensions of psychological problems that involve fear, worry, depression, and others kinds of human misery. These emotions are a common part of life, of course, and like all dimensions of psychological problems, they lie on continua. To reiterate a key point, one can experience anything from slight to extreme levels of internalizing problems, and those problems negatively impact our well-being, social relationships, employment, and income to varying degrees.[1,2]

The various dimensions described in this chapter are correlated, of course. They overlap with one another—to the extent that they can be said to define the second-order dimension of internalizing problems. To provide a heuristic framework, I have subgrouped the internalizing dimensions into subsets that seem to have important characteristics in common. For example, the first section here is headed "Fears and Panic Attacks," based both on data that the several correlated dimensions grouped under that rubric are highly correlated and on the assumption that they are similar in important ways. These subsets of dimensions should not be overinterpreted, however, as a great deal remains to be learned from comprehensive empirical studies about the best ways to organize the dimensions of psychological problems.

Fears and Panic Attacks

Human beings have evolved brain mechanisms that allow us to fear things and situations that pose threats to our physical survival. In some cases, however, we fear things or situations much more than the danger they actually pose to us. In that sense, they are "irrational" fears. We experience such fears on a continuum, but at the extreme end of the dimension, the object or situation immediately provokes fear to the extent that the stimulus must be either avoided or endured with distress. Often, these strong fear responses are accompanied by physiological arousal, such as sweating, a pounding heart, or difficulty breathing. There are three different dimensions of such fears: specific fears, agoraphobic fears, and panic attacks.

Specific Fears

These are fear responses to a specific physical object or situation to an extent that is not justified by their actual dangerousness. Commonly feared stimuli include heights, insects and other animals, blood, hypodermic injections, physicians and dentists, and automobiles. Persons differ continuously in the number of objects or situations that elicit fear, the consistency with which these things cause fear, and the extent to which the fear is distressing and interferes with their life functioning. For example, some persons are hardly bothered by being in safe places that are high above the ground, others are mildly uncomfortable in such high places, and still others are intensely afraid of heights. They may be unable to hold jobs that require being high above the ground, such as carpentry; may decline jobs working in offices on high floors; or may be unable to travel over high bridges, even when taking alternative routes would be longer and less efficient. Other specific fears, such as extreme fears of medical or dental procedures, can be intense enough to result in life-threatening avoidance of vaccinations or necessary procedures.

Agoraphobic Fears

Agoraphobic fears get their name from *agora*, the Greek word for a city's central public space and market. Such fears do not only occur in literal marketplaces but also occur in situations outside the person's home or "safe zone." Importantly, fear responses to such situations often do not occur, however, if the individual is accompanied by a partner, friend, or other "safe figure." This is quite different from specific fears, which are not typically allayed by the presence of others. Agoraphobic fears can be triggered simply by being even short distances outside the home alone. In some cases, individuals may be essentially home bound because of their intense agoraphobic fear, particularly if they do not have a "safe" partner to accompany them outside. In other cases, the fear occurs primarily when in public and *open spaces*, such as in fields, open-air gathering places, or parking lots. In contrast, the fear can also be elicited in *enclosed places* from which they might have difficulty getting help or leaving quickly if they experience fear. This includes being in tunnels, theaters, shops, any form of transportation, crowds or standing in line, or being on a bridge or in an elevator. The dimension of agoraphobic fear is defined by the number of situations in which the fear is evoked and the frequency and intensity of the fear.

Panic Attacks

A panic attack is a sudden and often very intense experience of fear that reaches full intensity within about 10 minutes. These attacks are like intense phobic reactions, except that panic attacks occur without warning and *not* in the presence of a feared object or situation. In addition to the conscious experience of fear, individuals having a panic attack often experience a hurricane of physiological arousal: a pounding increase in heartbeat, chest pain or discomfort, dizzy lightheadedness, sweating, trembling or shaking, shortness of breath or a sensation of smothering, choking, nausea or abdominal pain, numbness or tingling sensations, and chills or hot flushes. Individuals having panic attacks sometimes also experience unnerving feelings of depersonalization or derealization, which are described in Chapter 5. In describing the experience of their first panic attack, people sometimes say that they thought they were going crazy, had come unhinged, or were going to die. Panic attacks are often linked to agoraphobic fears, as some people become agoraphobic because they are afraid of having distressing and embarrassing panic attacks when they are alone and away from their safe place.

Because the physiological aspects of panic attacks are similar to the signs of a heart attack, persons experiencing a panic attack often go to an emergency room thinking they are having a heart attack. As a result, medical personnel in emergency rooms routinely ask questions to determine if the person is experiencing a panic attack rather than a heart attack. Panic attacks are relatively common experiences, and they can occur as isolated events that are not repeated. About 2–5% of people in the general population say they have experienced a panic attack during the past 12 months.[3,4] Some of these persons experience frequently repeated attacks, and over time they usually develop uncomfortable levels of worry about having their next panic attack.

Worry–Misery Problems

Unlike the internalizing problems just discussed, the various dimensions of internalizing problems described in this section do not involve acute fear but, rather, reflect less specific generalized worry, nervousness, tension, and unhappiness, which can either be long-lasting or wax and wane in episodes that last days, weeks, or months. Several such dimensions of psychological problems are grouped together in this section because they are correlated with one another. Among other things, this means that it is common to experience varying combinations of the specific problems from more than one of these dimensions.

Generalized Anxiety

A number of correlated specific psychological problems define this dimension of psychological problems. They cause problems for the person when they are both more frequent and more intense than expected given the realities of the person's situation and cause distress or impaired functioning. Widespread worries that many things are not going well and will not go well in the future are a cardinal feature of this dimension. These worries are difficult or impossible for the individual to voluntarily control. These pessimistic worries may be about friendships, spousal relationships, work, finances, and real or imagined dangers. This dimension also includes having subjective feelings of nervousness, sometimes including uncomfortable tingling feelings or "pins and needles" under the skin. Individuals may similarly feel keyed up, on edge, jumpy, or be easily startled. They may experience muscle tension or soreness and find it difficult or impossible to relax. They may feel restless or pace or move in agitated ways, and they may experience insomnia—difficulty falling asleep or staying asleep. Some persons with high levels of generalized anxiety find it difficult to concentrate and make decisions, and they sometimes feel that their mind has gone blank.

Health Worries

This dimension of psychological problems also involves unrealistic worry, but in this case it is worry about one's physical health. The correlated worries that define this dimension include frequent and exaggerated worries about their physical health in the absence of medical evidence of an actual health problem. They are easily alarmed by anything that might indicate that they have a health problem, such as a pain or feeling tired. When they learn that someone nearby may have a contagious illness, they may worry and go to exaggerated lengths to avoid the contagious person. They may be preoccupied with their health concerns, spend a lot of time focusing on them, and frequently check for symptoms. They may frequently talk about their health problems, often in dramatic ways; in earlier times, they were referred to uncharitably as "hypochondriacs." The person may experience pain or other bodily symptoms that cannot be explained by physicians. The fact that pain is quite common among persons who meet criteria for most DSM mental disorders complicates our understanding of this dimension.[5]

Individuals with high levels of health anxiety are often distressed by their worries, and their preoccupation with their health alienates friends and families. They often have problems keeping jobs because they miss work because of appointments with physicians and may bother coworkers with their frequent complaints and worries about their health. Furthermore, health worries can ironically harm the individual's health. Some persons who are excessively worried about their health overuse potentially dangerous medical services and treatments. They may "shop" for physicians who will provide the medications they want, often taking dangerous combinations of medications prescribed by multiple physicians. In some cases, they even talk surgeons into performing medically unjustified surgical procedures by complaining repeatedly and intensely about their pain and discomfort.

Depression

The problems of mood and "vegetative" functions—sleeping, eating, and other functions needed for the maintenance of life—that constitute the dimension of depression are common and are often very distressing and impairing. This dimension of psychological problems is the basis for the diagnosis of major depression in DSM. That is, the specific psychological problems that define this dimension are considered to be symptoms of major depression. Dysphoria, or intense sadness, that lasts for more than brief periods is a common part of this dimension. Some persons experience anhedonia, meaning a decreased interest in nearly all enjoyable activities, reduced experience of pleasure, and may have reduced motivation to even seek positive and pleasurable experiences. Some individuals blame themselves in exaggerated and unrealistic ways for bad things that have happened to themselves or others. For example, a person who loses their job as a clerk because the company where the person works closes its office during a recession may unreasonably believe that it was their incompetence alone that led to the closure. Persons may also experience difficulty concentrating and making decisions. Some individuals may experience less energy and more fatigue than they did before the episode of depressive problems began. Their motor movements and their thinking and speech may be slowed. They may sleep more than is usual for them, or they may experience the opposite—insomnia. They may experience a loss of appetite and lose weight without trying to do so, or they may experience the opposite—increased appetite and unintended weight gain. They may feel hopeless and not believe that things will ever get better in the future. They may think about death, wish they were dead, or even plan or attempt suicide. These correlated problems of depression are often, but not always, accompanied by low self-esteem, which is described later in this chapter when presenting the related dimension of rejection sensitivity.

Depression problems can be persistent, but usually they are not. Rather, depression typically comes and goes in episodes that last a couple of weeks to several months. Fortunately, the majority of people who experience an episode of intense depression will only do so once in their lifetimes.[6] People in the general population who experience a first episode of depression in which they meet DSM criteria have about a 15% chance of experiencing another episode within 5 years, with the chances of another episode increasing to about 25% within 10 years and about 40% within 20 years.[7]

Sluggish Cognitive Tempo

The problems that define this hypothesized dimension can interfere with school and work performance.[8] It is possible that this dimension will eventually be thought of as part of the depression dimension based on its high correlation with depression and because many of the defining specific problems are similar to depressive problems. Nonetheless, there is evidence that this should be considered to be an independent dimension.[8] Sluggish cognitive tempo is defined by the number and severity of a number of specific problems: Some people with these problems move slowly and sluggishly. They may be apathetic and have little motivation to do anything constructive. They may have trouble staying alert or awake during the day. They dawdle, procrastinate, and work inefficiently. They frequently get lost in their daydreams, stare into space, and appear to be confused about what is going on. When speaking or working, they may often lose their train of thought. They process information slowly and often take a long time to answer questions. More research is needed to decide how these problems should best be understood.

Post-Traumatic Stress Reactions

When people experience highly stressful events, their emotions, cognition, and behavior understandably can change. These changes may be immediate, but sometimes they do not appear until weeks or months later. In DSM, these changes are referred to as PTSD when severe. The traumatic stressful events that sometimes give rise to these problems include experiencing sexual or other kinds of physical abuse, experiencing actual or threatened violence, causing or witnessing someone's injury or death, narrowly avoiding one's own death in a motor vehicle accident or other situation, and learning that a relative or close friend was exposed to a trauma. Soldiers and first responders are particularly likely to experience such traumatic stress, but traumatic stressful events can happen to anyone. Some persons who experience these problems after traumatic stress improve within a matter of months, but in the absence of help, post-traumatic problems can last for years,

It is important to keep several issues in mind when considering post-traumatic stress reactions. First, many of the psychological problems that commonly emerge following traumatic stress also are found in individuals who have not experienced traumatic stress. That is, they are problems that are described elsewhere in this chapter as parts of their own dimensions of psychological problems. Second, traumatic stress can give rise to other dimensions of problems in addition to, or instead of, the stress reactions described here. Third, it is important to understand that stressful events are not always followed by psychological problems. Persons who experience stressful events should not believe that they will necessarily experience maladaptive changes in their emotions and cognitions, as it certainly does not always happen. Nonetheless, persons who experience highly stressful events are at increased risk for the problems discussed next.

Persons exposed to traumatic stress often become hypervigilant regarding cues related to the trauma. They may experience what is termed dissociative amnesia (i.e., an inability to recall aspects of the traumatic event, and sometimes even their own name and address), which is discussed in Chapter 5. Unfortunately, they may experience upsetting memories, nightmares, or flashbacks. Cues that remind the individual of the trauma often trigger distressing changes in emotion, perceptions, or physiological arousal. As a result, the individual often actively avoids reminders of the trauma to prevent these reactions.

Because stress can cause many kinds of psychological problems, it is inevitable that post-traumatic stress reactions can be quite broad. Many of the problems that accompany these reactions to traumatic stress are discussed as part of other dimensions elsewhere in this chapter and in Chapters 4 and 5. They include depressive problems— dysphoria, anhedonia, hopeless pessimism about the future, a negative view of oneself, exaggerated blame of oneself for the traumatic event, difficulty concentrating, insomnia, and intentional self-harm and suicidal behavior—but also irritability, physical aggression, antisocial behavior, substance abuse, reckless disregard for the safety of oneself, feeling detached or estranged from others, and paranoid suspiciousness (i.e., believing that no one is trustworthy).[9–11]

Some of the problems seen in persons who experience traumatic stress may be pre-existing characteristics of the individual. Indeed, they may be characteristics that are associated with an increased likelihood of people either experiencing traumatic stress or being vulnerable to experiencing problems following stress, rather than being psychological problems *caused* by the stress. For example, people who are characteristically irritable may be more likely to provoke traumatic physical assaults. This is an important theoretical issue that is addressed later in the book when I discuss "transactions" with the environment, but to persons experiencing psychological problems after traumatic stress, this point is not relevant to their need for help.

Social Anxiety and Dependence

The two dimensions of psychological problems described in this section both involve anxiety in social contexts. One dimension focuses on anxiety about being rejected by others, and the other focuses on fears of physical harm if not protected by others. These putative dimensions capture problems that are treated in the DSM as diagnoses of social anxiety disorder, avoidant personality, separation anxiety disorder, and dependent personality disorder.

Rejection Sensitivity

Some persons are easily and frequently upset by real or imagined criticism from others—they are very sensitive to any sign of disapproval or rejection. As a result of this rejection sensitivity, they may be unassertive and reluctant to disagree with others because of fear of disapproval or rejection by them. They may lack self-direction, and their opinions and behavior may be easily influenced by others. Because of their sensitivity to disapproval, they may be anxious about performing any skill in front of others, including public speaking. Similarly, they may avoid social situations in which they might be evaluated, such as working as part of a team. They may be anxious about situations in which they need to interact with unfamiliar people and may be reluctant to become involved in new social relationships unless they are confident of being liked. They often prefer to be unnoticed and are uncomfortable being the center of attention. They may particularly fear being viewed by others when they are exhibiting signs of anxiety, such as flushing, because they do not want to be criticized for being anxious. Not surprisingly, extreme social anxiety is often associated with impaired social relationships and feelings of loneliness.[12] In the DSM, this dimension forms the basis of the categorical diagnoses of both social anxiety disorder and avoidant personality disorder, which are very similar.

Social Dependence and Separation Anxiety

The specific psychological problems that define this dimension are considered in the DSM to be the symptoms of the diagnoses of separation anxiety disorder, particularly in children and adolescents, and dependent personality disorder in adults. Note that these problems can only be understood in terms of the person's relationship with a trusted figure to whom the person is attached. The common thread is fear of harm unless the attachment figure is there to protect them. The dimension of social dependence/separation anxiety is defined by the following correlated problems. Some people do not want to be self-sufficient and want an attachment figure to take care of them and be responsible for them, even when they reach adulthood. They may make extreme efforts to force the trusted attachment figure to take care of them, such as becoming very upset or threatening suicide if the attachment figure threatens to leave. If the relationship with the caring attachment figure does end, they urgently replace the attachment figure with a new one. Some persons feel frightened or uncomfortable when left alone to care for themselves. They may have difficulty making decisions on their own without the attachment figure. Some persons feel anxious when separation from the caring attachment figure is expected to happen or actually occurs. They may experience headaches, stomachaches, nausea, or vomiting when separation from the attachment figure occurs or is anticipated. They may worry that something bad will cause them to be separated from the attachment figure (e.g., getting lost, being kidnapped, or the attachment figure will have an illness or accident), or they may experience repeated nightmares about being separated from the attachment figure. Especially in childhood or adolescence, persons who experience separation anxiety may be reluctant, or even refuse, to go to school or elsewhere that would require separation from the attachment figure. In addition, the individual may refuse to go to sleep without the attachment figure in bed with them or nearby.

Borderline Emotional Instability

The dimension of borderline emotional instability is defined by correlated problems that correspond to some of the symptoms that define the binary diagnosis of borderline personality disorder in DSM. There are reasons to think of borderline emotional instability as being closely related to both internalizing and externalizing dimensions. On the one hand, the dimension of borderline emotional instability is included in this chapter on internalizing problems because it is very strongly correlated with problems of anxiety and depression, with more than 80% of adults who meet DSM diagnostic criteria for borderline personality disorder also meeting criteria for an anxiety disorder or depression at some time during their lives.[13] On the other hand, borderline emotional instability is strongly associated with the misuse of psychoactive substances, which is considered to be part of the externalizing domain.[13] Complicating the picture for borderline emotional instability, persons high on this dimension often display schizotypal problems, which are discussed in Chapter 5.[13]

Borderline emotional problems were initially thought to be highly persistent and unchanging, but there is evidence that they often fluctuate in episodes, which frequently co-occur with episodes of depression.[14] The problems that define borderline emotional instability include unstable and frequently changing emotions. Some individuals experience frequent, uncontrolled, intense, and inappropriate anger that is out of proportion to the situation. Persons with these problems tend to have an unstable self-concept and a shaky sense of their identity, meaning that their own sense of who they are and what they are like is unclear to themselves and often changes. They could think of themselves as intelligent, self-reliant, and successful at one moment but be convinced that they are weak and utterly stupid failures an hour later, with little justification for the frequent shifts back and forth between these extremes. In interpersonal relationships, they may similarly alternate between idealizing and adoring their partner and their friends to demeaning or even hating them. Some individuals with borderline problems experience paranoid thoughts that other people are "out to get them" or working against their interests. They may worry frequently about the infidelity of their partner without any cause. Some individuals with such problems may often experience feelings of emptiness and boredom. When they are upset, they may impulsively engage in self-harm, such as cutting or burning themselves, and make suicidal threats and engage in suicidal gestures that are unlikely to be fatal. In addition, problems of borderline emotional instability are often accompanied by problems of social dependence, including fear of being abandoned by one's partner or friends and making frantic efforts to avoid abandonment by others. With the exception of substance use problems, borderline emotional problems are more strongly associated with being homeless compared with any other psychological problem.[15,16]

References

1. Comer JS, Blanco C, Hasin DS, et al. Health-related quality of life across the anxiety disorders: Results from the National Epidemiologic Survey on Alcohol and Related Conditions (NESARC). *Journal of Clinical Psychiatry*. 2011;72(1):43–50.

2. Hellerstein DJ, Agosti V, Bosi M, Black SR. Impairment in psychosocial functioning associated with dysthymic disorder in the NESARC study. *Journal of Affective Disorders.* 2010;127(1–3):84–88.

3. de Jonge P, Roest AM, Lim CCW, et al. Cross-national epidemiology of panic disorder and panic attacks in the world mental health surveys. *Depression and Anxiety.* 2016;33(12):1155–1177.

4. Nay W, Brown R, Roberson-Nay R. Longitudinal course of panic disorder with and without agoraphobia using the National Epidemiologic Survey on Alcohol and Related Conditions (NESARC). *Psychiatry Research.* 2013;208(1):54–61.

5. Viana MC, Lim CCW, Pereira FG, et al. Previous mental disorders and subsequent onset of chronic back or neck pain: Findings from 19 countries. *Journal of Pain.* 2018;19(1):99–110.

6. Monroe SM, Anderson SF, Harkness KL. Life stress and major depression: The mysteries of recurrences. *Psychological Review.* 2019;126(6):791–816.

7. Nuggerud-Galeas S, Suescun LSB, Torrijo NB, et al. Analysis of depressive episodes, their recurrence and pharmacologic treatment in primary care patients: A retrospective descriptive study. *PLoS One.* 2020;15(5):e233454.

8. Becker SP, Leopold DR, Burns GL, et al. The internal, external, and diagnostic validity of sluggish cognitive tempo: A meta-analysis and critical review. *Journal of the American Academy of Child and Adolescent Psychiatry.* 2016;55(3):163–178.

9. Kessler RC, Galea S, Gruber MJ, Sampson NA, Ursano RJ, Wessely S. Trends in mental illness and suicidality after Hurricane Katrina. *Molecular Psychiatry.* 2008;13(4):374–384.

10. Nock MK, Hwang I, Sampson NA, Kessler RC. Mental disorders, comorbidity and suicidal behavior: Results from the National Comorbidity Survey Replication. *Molecular Psychiatry.* 2010;15(8):868–876.

11. Ramsawh HJ, Fullerton CS, Mash HBH, et al. Risk for suicidal behaviors associated with PTSD, depression, and their comorbidity in the US Army. *Journal of Affective Disorders.* 2014;161:116–122.

12. Maes M, Nelemans SA, Danneel S, et al. Loneliness and social anxiety across childhood and adolescence: Multilevel meta-analyses of cross-sectional and longitudinal associations. *Developmental Psychology.* 2019;55(7):1548–1565.

13. Tomko RL, Trull TJ, Wood PK, Sher KJ. Characteristics of borderline personality disorder in a community sample: Comorbidity, treatment utilization, and general functioning. *Journal of Personality Disorders.* 2014;28(5):734–750.

14. Gunderson JG, Morey LC, Stout RL, et al. Major depressive disorder and borderline personality disorder revisited: Longitudinal interactions. *Journal of Clinical Psychiatry.* 2004;65(8):1049–1056.

15. Tsai J. Lifetime and 1-year prevalence of homelessness in the US population: Results from the National Epidemiologic Survey on Alcohol and Related Conditions–III. *Journal of Public Health.* 2018;40(1):65–74.

16. Krausz RM, Strehlau V, Schuetz C. Homeless, poor, and hopeless—Substance use, mental illness and homelessness: Research from the US and Canada. *Suchttherapie.* 2016;17(3):131–136.

4

Dimensions of Externalizing Problems

Unlike the internalizing problems discussed in Chapter 3, externalizing problems are not defined by the experience of inherently distressing emotions such as anxiety or sadness. Rather, they are defined by patterns of behavior that interfere with living a successful and satisfying life. People with high levels of externalizing problems are often very distressed, but they are mostly distressed by the *consequences* of their actions. Their behaviors interfere with functioning in school, work, and other settings; alienate peers and family members; and can lead to serious social consequences, such as being fired from employment or incarceration.

Another reason for distinguishing between internalizing and externalizing problems is that externalizing problems are often more persistent than internalizing problems, which are more likely to come and go in discrete episodes. This is only a relative difference, however, as externalizing problems also wax (get worse for a while) and wane (get better for a while) over time, sometimes ceasing altogether.[1]

Externalizing problems are distinguished from other kinds of psychological problems partly for these conceptual reasons but primarily based on empirical patterns of correlations among them. That is, the specific problems that define each dimension of externalizing problems are highly correlated with one another, and the several externalizing dimensions described in this chapter are highly correlated with one another.[2-4] Although externalizing dimensions are also correlated with internalizing and other dimensions of psychological problems, they are less correlated with them than with one another. That complex statement simply means that these birds of a feather flock together based on their correlations (i.e., the frequency of their co-occurrence).

Problems of Inattention and Hyperactivity–Impulsivity

The first two externalizing dimensions described in this chapter are the basis for the *Diagnostic and Statistical Manual of Mental Disorders* (DSM) diagnostic category of attention-deficit/hyperactivity disorder (ADHD).[5] These problems begin in childhood, improve over the course of development, but sometimes persist into adulthood. In the DSM, the binary diagnosis of ADHD is given to persons who display at least six of the nine problems of inattention described in this chapter, or six of the nine problems of hyperactivity–impulsivity, or both. These problems must cause distress or impaired functioning and must have been present for at least 6 months to meet criteria for the DSM diagnosis, although these problems are usually far more enduring than that.

Inattention

The inattention dimension of problems involves difficulties attending to task-related stimuli, remembering important things, and dealing with the demands of life in an organized manner. Almost everyone forgets and fails to attend at times—these are ubiquitous human failings—but impairment can result when the lack of attention and disorganization are frequent and extreme enough to interfere with accurately completing important tasks such as schoolwork and work. Specifically, some people find it difficult to pay attention for a sustained period of time during lectures, work tasks, conversations, or when reading. They do not listen carefully when spoken to directly, often missing important instructions for completing tasks in school or at work. They may be distracted frequently by extraneous stimuli in their environments or may be distracted by their own thoughts when attempting to attend. When working on tasks, some individuals fail to pay close attention to details and make careless mistakes at home, school, or work. Individuals high on the inattention dimension often dislike tasks that require sustained mental effort and avoid them as a result. They have difficulty organizing activities; do messy work; and frequently do not finish schoolwork, chores, or other work in a reasonable amount of time. Persons with high levels of inattention are often disorganized and may fail to turn in their work, and they lose things that are necessary for their work or activities, such as books, assignments, pencils, tools, wallets, keys, eyeglasses, and mobile telephones. They are often forgetful in their daily activities, such as when doing chores, running errands, paying bills, or keeping appointments.[5]

When middle-school children with problems of inattention are faced with the task of completing nightly homework in four school subjects, the challenge of writing down the assignments and getting those assignments home along with the books needed for the homework, remembering to do the homework that night and put it in their backpack, remembering to take their backpack to school, listening to teachers when they tell them to turn in their homework, and then actually turning it in is often too much to manage. Different versions of the same story could be told about the interference of inattention problems with success from kindergarten through college and into jobs.[6-8]

It is worth noting that persons who exhibit such problems are usually able to pay attention and organize their activities when the task is inherently interesting or important to them or when they are given strong incentives to pay attention.[9] In contrast, they often fail to pay attention when they find the task to be routine or boring. Thus, the same persons who are very inattentive and disorganized in school or at a job that they do not like may be highly attentive to videogames or activities that they enjoy. That is, even persons with high levels of attention problems *can* pay attention, but often they do not pay attention when performing the kinds of important tasks required at school or work that they find boring.[9] This statement absolutely should not lead us to *blame* persons with attention problems for not trying hard enough with the routine demands of school and work. Inattention is a complex process that involves both cognitive and motivational processes, and persons with higher levels of inattention problems just have a more difficult time paying attention to things that are not inherently interesting than most other persons.

Hyperactivity–Impulsivity

Persons with high levels of attention problems often, but not always, also have problems involving motor activity and impulsive behavior. The term *hyperactivity–impulsivity* refers a dimension defined by higher than average levels of motor activity and impulsive behavior that interferes with task performance and social functioning and is associated with an increased risk of physical injury.[5] People who are extreme on the hyperactivity–impulsivity dimension are physically active and behave in impulsive ways. They may seem to be always "on the go" and act like they are "driven by a motor inside" that keeps them in motion. During childhood, they run around more than most children or climb on things in situations in which it is inappropriate to do so. This particular aspect of hyperactivity usually declines with age, but adults may experience subjective feelings of restlessness when they are expected to be still. People who are extreme on the hyperactivity–impulsivity dimension often find it difficult to stay seated when it is necessary for school, work, or other quiet activities. When they are required to be seated, they often fidget or squirm and are likely to leave their seat in situations in which remaining seated is expected, such as in school classrooms. Especially during childhood, they may seem to be unable to play or engage in leisure activities quietly. Persons who are high on this dimension also often talk excessively. They may blurt out answers before the question has been completed, and they often have difficulty waiting for their turn in games or conversations and find it difficult to wait in lines. They may interrupt or intrude on others, such as by butting into conversations, games, or activities when not invited. High levels of hyperactivity–impulsivity can be very challenging in school, work, and social situations.[6,10] As children grow older, their hyperactivity–impulsivity problems decline considerably on average, but their inattention problems decline to a lesser extent.[6] This means that some adults continue to be impaired by inattention problems that they have had all their lives.[11,12]

Impairment Associated with ADHD Problems

At first blush, inattention and hyperactivity–impulsivity seem like pretty minor issues as psychological problems go, but the effects on meeting life's demands can sometimes be devastating. It has taken both the public and the mental health field a long time to recognize how serious high levels of inattention and hyperactivity can sometimes be for children, adolescents, and adults. This is probably because we all let our attention drift, lose our pens, and get restless in boring situations. These are common glitches in human behavior, particularly among children, and it is hard to take them seriously. Nonetheless, higher than average levels of the distraction and disorganization associated with inattention problems and the highly impulsive and active behavior associated with hyperactivity–impulsivity problems often play havoc with meeting the demands of life.

One difficulty in seeing how much impairment is associated with ADHD problems comes from the fact that ADHD frequently co-occurs with other dimensions of psychological problems.[4] For this reason, I have devoted a good bit of my own research time to teasing apart the contribution of ADHD and other correlated problems to impaired functioning in children, partly just to be sure that ADHD was impairing enough by itself to consider interventions to reduce those problems. We and many other teams of researchers found that high levels of ADHD problems, after statistically controlling for intelligence and other co-occurring psychological problems, create significant problems in interactions with peers and in meeting the academic demands of the classroom and are associated with increased risk of accidental injuries, including fatal injuries.[5,10,13,14] On average, children with high levels of ADHD problems also will have lower educational and occupational attainment in adulthood.[15–17] They are more likely to default on debts and less likely to earn a living in stable and well-paid occupations.[18] In addition, persons with ADHD problems are at somewhat increased risk for depression and suicidal behavior,[19] particularly when their economic situations deteriorate.[18]

Not everyone with ADHD problems in childhood has difficulties in adulthood, of course. Many are very successful and happy. Although ADHD is independently associated with impaired functioning during childhood and adolescence, parents can be guardedly optimistic about the adult outcomes of children who exhibit *only* ADHD problems during both childhood and adolescence.[6] Their residual ADHD symptoms in adulthood may still cause problems and require adjustments, and medication or other interventions may be needed, but childhood ADHD by itself does not always lead to an unsuccessful adult life. The adult outcomes of children with ADHD problems are much worse if they have co-occurring childhood oppositional–defiant and conduct problems (described in the section).[13,20,21] When they grow up, these children are more likely to exhibit antisocial and borderline problems, depression and suicidal behavior,[19,22] and substance abuse during adulthood.[23,24]

Oppositional and Antisocial Behavior

The several dimensions of externalizing problems that I describe here cause distress and dysfunction by pitting the individual against others. Oppositional and antisocial behaviors annoy, alienate, and sometimes humiliate and even harm other people. For most of us, it is more difficult to feel sympathy for persons who engage in these behaviors than for people who suffer from anxiety or depression. Furthermore, it is easy to caricature persons who engage in these behaviors as being heartless villains. Such views are not entirely unfounded in some cases, but it is important to keep in mind that persons who engage in high levels of antagonistic and antisocial behavior are fully human. They want to be loved and they love others to the extent that they can. They want to succeed in life and they often are made miserable by the consequences of their behavior, including the loss of personal relationships and employment, incarceration, and homelessness. Remember that their problem behaviors arise in ordinary ways, just like any other psychological problem. That does not mean that they should not be held accountable for their crimes, but we should remember that they did not ask to have externalizing problems.

Although externalizing problems have been studied intensively for many years, we are still a long way from fully understanding them. One issue is that the externalizing dimensions that have emerged from empirical studies do not map well onto binary DSM diagnostic categories. This is mostly the case because DSM diagnostic categories are based on varying and heterogeneous admixtures of the dimensions described in this chapter. For example, as discussed later in this chapter, some of the children and adolescents who meet diagnostic criteria for conduct disorder and some of the adults who meet diagnostic criteria for antisocial personality disorder display only reactive antisocial behaviors, some display only proactive antisocial behaviors, and some engage in both kinds of behaviors. These are a mixed bag of problems with at least partly different causes.[25]

Oppositional–Defiant Behavior

From childhood through adulthood, people high on this dimension are often touchy and irritable, as shown in being easily annoyed, frustrated, offended, and provoked. They blame others for their misdeeds and deny responsibility for their mistakes and misbehaviors. They often throw screaming, stomping temper tantrums—mostly in childhood, but sometimes during adulthood—and experience bouts of intense anger when they are criticized, frustrated, or cannot have their way. Some persons with these problems stubbornly defy and oppose legitimate and appropriate instructions from persons in roles of authority. When a parent tells a highly oppositional child to pick up his dirty clothes, the response is often a belligerently defiant "no!" If the parent insists, the child may argue angrily and throw a temper tantrum. Highly oppositional individuals often behave in spiteful, malicious, and mean ways toward others, particularly when they are annoyed or angry with them. They often hold vindictive grudges and seek revenge for wrongs that they believe were unjustly inflicted on them by others. They portray themselves as the victims of other people's misbehaviors and rarely admit to instigating fights and other altercations.

The tendency to engage in oppositional and defiant problems is typically an enduring trait-like characteristic of the individual, but the irritable and oppositional behaviors are not present every minute of every day and may erupt only during bouts of anger or other negative emotions. The difficulty is that these bouts of negative emotion are often frequent, being easily precipitated by frustrations, threats, or other provocations for which the individual has a very low tolerance.

Persons who display four or more such problem behaviors for at least 6 months meet the DSM's diagnostic criteria for the diagnosis of oppositional defiant disorder. Thirty years ago, this diagnosis was added to an earlier edition of the DSM to give a diagnosis to misbehaving children whose parents sought help from psychologists but who did not meet criteria for any other mental disorder. Oppositional defiant disorder was thought at that time be a relatively minor problem. Later, it became clear that many children and adolescents who behave in oppositional and defiant ways go on to develop the more serious problems that define the DSM diagnosis of conduct disorder. It also became clear that some of the children who meet criteria for conduct disorder subsequently meet diagnostic criteria for the very serious diagnosis of antisocial personality disorder during adulthood (both described later in this chapter).[26]

Thus, oppositional–defiant problems are important because of their role as a developmental precursor to serious antisocial problems in adulthood—particularly when they co-occur with the problems that define ADHD, which they often do. Nonetheless, it is now clear that oppositional–defiant behaviors by themselves seriously impair social functioning, both during childhood and into adolescence and adulthood.[27,28] Children and adolescents who behave in highly oppositional–defiant ways are more than a handful for their parents and teachers, and they are frequently rejected by their peers as friends and playmates and often become the targets of aggression from their peers.[29]

Reactive Antisocial Behavior

This dimension often co-occurs with the irritable–defiant problems just described, but it may be different enough to distinguish as a separate dimension of psychological problems. Reactive aggression is defined by being easily provoked into either angry physical aggression against other people or nonaggressive acts, such as a toddler angrily taking another child's toy, an adolescent reacting with emotion-driven vandalism, or an adult angrily taking someone's stash of drugs. Persons who engage in high levels of reactive aggression appear to have little control over their emotions and aggressive actions at the time. Future research may suggest that reactive antisocial behavior is simply oppositional–defiant behavior that crosses the line from tantrums to antisocial acts, but we currently do not have enough evidence to decide.

Proactive Antisocial Behavior

This dimension describes a pattern of antisocial behavior that, unlike reactive antisocial behavior, does not occur only when the person is angry or upset. This kind of antisocial behavior is thus termed proactive instead of reactive, but it is not proactive in the sense of always being committed after careful planning. Indeed, there often is an impulsive and opportunistic quality to proactive antisocial behavior. The distinction is based on the extent to which the antisocial behavior is committed only during bouts of anger—such as reactively hitting a person in a bar who speaks to one's date—as opposed to calmly following a woman seen on the street to her home and breaking in for the purpose of stealing her possessions or raping her. Not all proactive antisocial behaviors are as serious and harmful to others as this example, however. Some teenagers dislike following rules set by adults and commit relatively minor "status offenses" not during the heat of emotion. Status offenses are actions that are legal for adults but not for minors, such as truancy from school, violating family curfews, and running away from home.

It is important to keep in mind that reactive and proactive antisocial behavior are positively correlated. There are differences between reactive and proactive antisocial behavior,[30] and some persons almost exclusively engage in one or the other kind, but it is quite common for the same person to display both reactive and proactive antisocial behavior. Remember, psychological problems never come in separate silos. People very often display a mishmash of all kinds of problems, including antisocial behaviors.

Antisocial Behavior and Gangs

We can learn an important lesson about antisocial behavior by looking at membership in antisocial gangs. Gang members are disproportionally responsible for drug selling, assaults and murders, and other crimes by youth in many countries. Why do gangs exist? Are gangs organizations created by already antisocial youth or do gangs socialize their members into antisocial behavior? The answer is both. Youth who will later join gangs are already more antisocial than other youth, and their rates of antisocial behavior are accelerating even before they join gangs.[31] So already antisocial youth are the ones who join gangs. Once they are in a gang, however, there are additional sharp increases in their drug use, drug selling, vandalism, and violent behavior. When they leave the gang, those behaviors decline again. Thus, being in a gang appears to be a powerful environmental force that exacerbates already serious antisocial behavior.[31]

Psychopathic Behavior

Before discussing the DSM diagnoses that map—to a degree—onto reactive and proactive antisocial behavior, we should look at the concept of *psychopathy*.[32,33] It is probably better to think of this important construct not as a dimension of antisocial behavior but, rather, as a dimension of "personality characteristics" that both disposes some individuals to engage in antisocial behavior and moderates or worsens the severity of antisocial behavior. Nonetheless, although psychopathic characteristic are substantially correlated with antisocial behavior, they can be found in persons whose antisocial behavior is subtle or even technically legal, as in the case of highly self-serving business practices such as selling weight loss products that are known to be worthless.

As you read this section, keep in mind that like all dimensions of psychological problems, psychopathic characteristics are continuous, with many people exhibiting one or two of them and only a few people exhibiting all of these characteristic. There is no natural cutoff between "psychopathic" and "normal." It is all a matter of degree.

Psychopathic characteristics are diverse. They include acting in callous, selfish, and self-centered ways that show little regard for the safety and welfare of others, including the health and safety of their own children. Persons high on the psychopathy dimension are often irresponsible. Most of us work to make a living, pay our bills, and take care of our families, but highly psychopathic individuals tend not to do so. They are often absent from work and do not perform their duties carefully. They do not consistently pay their bills and are unlikely to pay their debts. Highly psychopathic individuals often lead parasitic lifestyles in which they selfishly convince others to support them and supply them with money for alcohol, drugs, and other needs. When this parasitic pattern is extreme, it can include actions such as pimping and taking most of the earnings of persons they coerce into prostitution. Psychopathic individuals are often impulsive in the sense of acting on the spur of the moment and not planning ahead. As a result, they move from one place to another frequently without thinking the move through and quit jobs before they have new ones. Consequently, they are often unemployed and homeless until they find the next victim to exploit.

Highly psychopathic individuals are often successful in taking advantage of others partly because they often behave in poised and socially dominant ways. They may be able to smoothly manipulate, deceive, or exploit others for their own personal gain. They are con artists in small and sometimes very serious ways. The people who scam vulnerable individuals by selling them unnecessary and shoddy roof repairs or by using internet scams to bleed their victim's life savings are often highly psychopathic. Frighteningly, some of these con artists are referred to as "high-functioning psychopaths" because they are well educated, well dressed, and present themselves in a positive light. They often use their positions as elected government officials or financial advisors to bamboozle vast amounts of money through bribes, Ponzi schemes, and other deceptions. Women who exhibit psychopathic characteristics are somewhat more likely than males to also behave in ways that are typical of the histrionic–narcissistic dimension of problems described later in this chapter. In particular, they may use their lively friendliness and seductive dress and behavior to manipulate others in antisocial ways.

Persons who are extreme in psychopathic behavior are often described as being *unemotional*. This does not mean that they are devoid of all emotions but, rather, they are unemotional in some very important ways. They may express concern for others, but they do so in ways that are glib, shallow, and insincere. They may coldly and unemotionally take advantage of others or hurt them physically. When they break the law or take advantage of other people, highly psychopathic individuals typically experience little or no guilt or remorse about their misdeeds. They show little real emotion in their reactions to the pain or misery of others. Because reactive and proactive patterns of antisocial behavior often co-occur, however, it is not uncommon for persons with many psychopathic traits to be very emotional in the sense of being irritable, hostile, and easily losing their temper and engaging in reactive violence.

Some individuals high on the psychopathy continuum seek out and enjoy excitement, thrills, and taking risks, and they display little fear regarding their own personal safety. Indeed, some experts believe that such fearlessness is a core characteristic of psychopathic behavior.[34] Fearlessness is important not only because fear plays an adaptive role in keeping us from engaging in dangerous activities but also because it is involved in learning to avoid the painful and otherwise adverse consequences of our actions. When punished, highly psychopathic individuals may not learn to stop misbehaving because they do not fear future punishments. One interesting alternative theory[35,36] suggests that this fearlessness is not the result of deficits in the brain systems that operate during fear but, rather, the result of the attention problems that many persons who are high in psychopathy exhibit. That is, persons high in psychopathy may be fearless only because they do not pay sufficient attention to signals of impending danger that make most people fearful. This inattention is not specific to dangerous stimuli; rather, it is a general problem of inattention of the sort described previously in this chapter. This observation is consistent with findings that the children who are most likely to grow up to exhibit antisocial behavior in adulthood are those with both attention deficits and oppositional–defiant and conduct problems.[37,38]

As is implied in the description of psychopathy, persons who are extreme on this dimension often engage in illegal activities. They often commit property crimes, including theft and fraud, but people with psychopathic characteristics are often aggressive as well. Beyond deliberately annoying, intimidating, and bullying others, they sometimes intentionally and unemotionally hurt others in physically and emotionally brutal ways, including rape, physical assaults, and homicide.[39] As noted at the beginning of this section, psychopathic characteristics can be thought of as exacerbating the severity of reactive and proactive antisocial behavior. Even compared to other convicted criminal offenders, psychopathic individuals begin their criminal careers at earlier ages, commit more criminal offenses per year, are more violent and sadistic, and are more likely to quickly resume their criminal behavior after release from prison.[40]

DSM Diagnostic Categories Associated with Antisocial Behavior

The DSM diagnostic categories that capture high and impairing levels of antisocial behaviors were designed for persons of different ages. Conduct disorder is the binary diagnosis given to children and adolescents who display at least 3 of 15 proactive and reactive antisocial behaviors. The antisocial behaviors that are most common in children and adolescents given the diagnosis of conduct disorder are bullying, starting fights, and lying to con others, but more serious antisocial behaviors, such as forced sex, burglary, mugging, and using a weapon, are not uncommon in adolescents with serious conduct problems.[41]

Beginning at age 18 years, persons can be given the binary DSM diagnosis of antisocial personality disorder if they (a) met criteria for conduct disorder by the age of 15 years and (b) exhibit at least four impairing problems during adulthood. This diagnosis is based on a mixture of both antisocial behaviors and psychopathic characteristics. One of the "symptoms" of antisocial personality disorder refers to a general disregard for laws and societal norms, which can be met by engaging in the specific proactive or reactive antisocial behaviors such as theft or forced sex. Two "symptoms" of antisocial personality disorder refer to specific proactive or reactive antisocial behaviors (e.g., lying to manipulate or con others and physical aggression). Nonetheless, the majority of the symptoms of antisocial personality disorder are not antisocial behaviors but are psychopathic characteristics: impulsivity, reckless disregard for the safety of self and others, consistent irresponsibility, dishonest manipulation of others for profit or self-amusement, and lack of guilt regarding antisocial actions. Again, psychopathy apparently moderates the severity of antisocial behavior. Capacity for guilt seems to be particularly important in this regard. The half of all persons who meet criteria for antisocial personality disorder who display little or no remorse over their misbehaviors are very likely to be violent, whereas the half who do show remorse engage mostly in nonviolent property crimes.[42]

Because the "symptoms" of the highly heterogeneous diagnosis of antisocial personality include both antisocial behaviors and psychopathic characteristics, some persons meet diagnostic criteria for antisocial personality disorder on the basis of their irresponsible and parasitic lifestyles but commit few actual crimes. Indeed, only about half of persons who meet criteria for antisocial personality disorder are ever charged with a crime.[43,44] This does not mean that the other half functions well. Whether they commit crimes or not, people who meet criteria for antisocial personality disorder have markedly disrupted personal and economic lives—including frequent unemployment, unhappy partner relationships and frequent divorces, and homelessness—and are at risk for serious accidental injuries that cause physical disabilities, being the victim of assault, and being infected with and spreading infections such as HIV and hepatitis C.[43] They suffer high rates of physical disability and tend to die prematurely due to illnesses, violence, drug overdoses, and suicide.[45-47]

As just noted, adults can only be given the DSM diagnosis of antisocial personality disorder if they previously met criteria for conduct disorder during childhood. A number of longitudinal studies have documented the strong developmental link between child and adolescent conduct problems and later antisocial personality disorder.[48] Their long antisocial "careers" are disproportionately important to society at large because highly antisocial persons are a small percentage of the population but account for 50% of all criminal convictions and comprise one-fourth of all welfare recipients.[49] Slightly less than half of those who meet criteria for conduct disorder continue to be antisocial enough to meet criteria for antisocial behavior,[50] but the ones who do make the lives of their victims miserable and are often just as miserable themselves.

Narcissistic–Histrionic Problems

The problems that define this dimension of impairing interpersonal behaviors are defined in the DSM as the "symptoms" of two different personality disorders—histrionic personality disorder and narcissistic personality disorder—but most evidence suggests that these problematic behaviors constitute a single dimension.[51-54] Persons who are extreme on this narcissistic–histrionic dimension feel unreasonably entitled to highly favorable treatment. They require excessive admiration from others. They expect others to do what they say, and they get upset if others do not do so. They often act in an arrogant and haughty manner and express their feelings and opinions in melodramatic, extreme, and exaggerated ways that are vague and lacking in detail. They believe that they are unique and superior to most other people. They identify themselves with high-status individuals and believe that only other special people can understand them, but they are nonetheless envious of other high-status people. They believe that anyone who dislikes them is just envious and jealous of them. They often interact with other people in inappropriately sexual and seductive ways, but they have difficulty achieving mature intimacy in relationships. Keep in mind that this is a continuum like all other dimensions of psychological problems. Few persons exhibit all of the specific problems just mentioned, but everyone falls somewhere on the histrionic–narcissistic dimension, from exhibiting none of these problems to exhibiting all of them.

Psychoactive Substance Use Problems

All of the many chemical substances that are *psychoactive* in the sense of altering our mood, cognition, energy, and behavior—from alcohol to heroin—are subject to misuse. Because they powerfully change how we feel, think, and behave, they can interfere with our adaptive behavior. In addition, it is not uncommon for persons who use psychoactive substances to become dependent on—addicted to—them. As a result, psychoactive substances are often used in ways that cause serious distress, impair life functioning, hurt innocent people, and cause high numbers of premature deaths.

This not to say that the use of psychoactive substances always causes problems for people. The great majority of occasional and low-level users of alcohol and marijuana would say that they use these substances without distress and impairment. Our focus in this chapter is on the harmful use of these substances, however. In this conversation, we must keep in mind that some of the worst harm associated with psychoactive substance use can be inflicted on users of illegal substances by criminal laws enacted in the name of the war on drugs. When these laws criminalize possession of small amounts of the psychoactive substances that are more often used by non-White persons, they can have disastrous consequences whether the intent of these laws is consciously racist or not.[55]

Three empirical facts frame our discussion of the harmful use of psychoactive substances. First, a proportion of first-time users of every kind of psychoactive substance progress to distressing and impairing substance use problems. Second, driving, working, and taking care of children when using alcohol, marijuana, or other psychoactive substances is associated with sharply increased risk for accidents that are often disabling or fatal to the user and to innocent persons.[56] Third, the use of most psychoactive substances is associated with risk of sudden and premature death. In terms of its impact on the population, the deadliest psychoactive drug is nicotine in tobacco. Daily tobacco smokers have a mortality rate that is three time higher than that of non-smokers, with more than 480,000 persons per year in the United States dying an average of 10 years earlier than non-smokers (https://www.cdc.gov/tobacco/data_statistics/fact_sheets/health_effects/tobacco_related_mortality/index.htm). These numbers are distressing, but they do not do justice to the genuinely horrible fact that millions of smokers, and persons who have to breathe their secondhand smoke, die painful deaths from chronic bronchitis and cancer of the trachea and lungs every year.

Nicotine is certainly not the only dangerous psychoactive substance, of course. An estimated 88,000 Americans die prematurely each year due to high levels alcohol consumption (https://www.niaaa.nih.gov/publications/brochures-and-fact-sheets/alcohol-facts-and-statistics). In addition, more than 67,000 people die each year in the United States from overdoses of opioid pain killers, stimulants, sedatives, tranquilizers, and inhalants (https://www.cdc.gov/drugoverdose/data/statedeaths.html).

Substance Abuse and Dependence

In this book, the dimension of *substance use problems* is defined by both the number of misused substances and the extent to which any psychoactive substance creates distress and dysfunction. In DSM-5, the new diagnostic category of *substance use disorder* combines what were previously considered to be the symptoms of *substance abuse* with the symptoms of *substance dependence* defined in previous editions of the DSM. Although the details differ considerably for each substance, people are said to *abuse* a psychoactive substance if they continue to use the substance despite the adverse consequences it has on their families or friends, on their school or work productivity, or in terms of promoting criminal behavior. The experience of substance dependence also differs from one psychoactive substance to another, but it has the common features of tolerance, cravings, and withdrawal. When a person develops tolerance to a substance, progressively larger amounts of the substance are needed to have the same effect. The person experiences intense cravings for the substance, and their need to use the substance may be more important than, and interfere with, their responsibilities to family, friends, and work. The person experiences uncomfortable withdrawal symptoms when the substance is not used. In the early stages of dependence, such withdrawal symptoms are relatively mild, but their intensity increases as the person becomes more dependent.

A major problem in studying and understanding the harm associated with substance use problems is that they so often occur with other psychological problems. Indeed, substance use problems are considered to be part of the externalizing domain because they frequently co-occur with antisocial behavior and other externalizing problems. DSM diagnoses of substance use disorders are far more common among persons with every externalizing dimension of psychological problems, but especially antisocial personality disorder.[57–59] Furthermore, substance use problems are more common in persons with problems of anxiety, depression, and personality disorders.[57,58,60,61]

Persons who are dependent on a substance spend large amounts of time obtaining and using the substance, and they may spend a considerable amount of time recovering from the effects of using the substance. They frequently keep a supply of the substance on hand, often hiding it from disapproving family members. They often spend more money on the substance than they can afford, and if necessary, persons dependent on psychoactive substances commit crimes or engage in prostitution to pay for the substance. Often, the person has tried unsuccessfully to reduce the amount of the substance used or to stop using it altogether many times. The person who is dependent on a substance may also find that they are cross-tolerant, meaning that they need larger doses of other substances to have the usual effect.[62]

Nicotine Dependence

Nicotine in tobacco is a powerfully addictive substance, with two-thirds of regular smokers being dependent.[63,64] In contrast, about one-fourth of people who regularly drink alcohol, about 20% of persons who use cocaine, and about 15% of persons who use marijuana are dependent.[64,65] The development of dependence on nicotine occurs gradually as more cigarettes are smoked on a daily basis and signs of craving and withdrawal become more frequent and intense when not smoking.[63]

Alcohol Dependence

In the case of alcohol, the individual not only drinks more as dependence develops but also may develop a narrow pattern of drinking that is mostly limited to a particular kind of alcohol. This rigid pattern of drinking serves to keep the individual (barely) functioning while drinking enough to avoid withdrawal symptoms. This pattern of drinking often does not vary much on workdays and holidays or when alone or with company.

Cocaine Dependence

The pattern of drug use associated with dependence on cocaine is very different from that of most psychoactive substances. Cocaine induces extreme euphoria and energy in many individuals. Few people use cocaine daily, but instead the dependent individual binges on frequent doses of cocaine for several hours to 24 hours or more, followed by crashing and abstaining from cocaine for several days. Highly dependent cocaine users binge once a week or more. They often use alcohol or other drugs to come down after the cocaine high, and they sometimes use marijuana, sedatives, or heroin to reduce the anxiety than can accompany binges. Between binges, the individual often experiences apathy and restlessness. Dependent users' thoughts are focused on the next binge, sometimes leading to ignoring nutrition, work, and the needs of family members. Just as not all users of alcohol become dependent, not all users of cocaine do so, but a large minority do.[66]

Heroin and Opioid Dependence

Heroin is a powerful drug with a high likelihood of dire consequences from its use. It is estimated that 300–500 people try heroin for the first time in the United States each day, and 30–50 users die of an overdose each day.[67] Among persons who try heroin for the first time, more than 40% become dependent on it.[67] More than 900,000 people in the United States use heroin and 1 million people misuse opioid pain relievers each year.[68] More than 47,000 people die of opioid overdose in the United States each year, making it the leading cause of accidental death, surpassing even death from motor vehicle accidents.[67]

Cannabis Abuse and Dependence

Many people use cannabis—often referred to as marijuana or pot—without harmful consequences, but it contains the psychoactive substance tetrahydrocannabinol (THC), which is one of many psychoactive substances that increase the risk of motor vehicle and other accidents.[69,70] Some teenagers and adults appear to abuse marijuana in the sense of using it instead of going to school or work, but it is not clear if these persons would be skipping school or work if they had never heard of or used pot. Still, the worrisome possibility is that smoking pot makes things worse at the very least.

It is clear, however, that some individuals—perhaps around 15%—become dependent on cannabis in the sense of developing tolerance and experiencing withdrawal symptoms when they cannot use it.[65] Now that cannabis has become legal for both medical and recreational use in many U.S. states, there has been a clear increase in the number of adults who use cannabis, although there has not been an increase in adolescent cannabis users to date.[71--73] Not enough information is available yet to know if this has led to an increase in the prevalence of cannabis abuse and dependence.[71-73] There is evidence that the increase in the potency of cannabis in the United States is associated with more frequent progression to dependence,[74] but this important topic needs further study. It is clear, however, that persons who begin using cannabis at earlier ages are more likely to develop cannabis use problems. This finding might mean that cannabis exposure is harmful to the developing brain, but it could mostly reflect the fact that youth with more externalizing problems are more likely to begin using all psychoactive substances at earlier ages.[61]

Two other inconclusive findings from research on cannabis use should give us pause for thought about cannabis use and encourage us to conduct stronger research. Women who use cannabis when pregnant are more likely to have children with psychological problems and thinner cerebral cortices in the brain than other women.[75,76] We cannot yet determine, however, if this is because exposure to THC during pregnancy influences prenatal brain development in harmful ways or if women who continue to use cannabis during pregnancy are different in ways that are the actual causes of the problems in their children. In addition, there is now clear evidence from many studies that youth who use cannabis more frequently are more likely to develop psychotic behavior.[77] This does not mean that cannabis use causes psychosis, of course, as persons disposed to later psychosis may simply be more likely to use cannabis as teenagers. Still there is worry that cannabis use could trigger the onset of psychotic behavior in people who are predisposed to it. One study statistically controlled for psychological problems prior to starting cannabis use, which strengthens the case for cannabis use increasing the risk for psychosis but certainly does not prove it.[78]

References

1. Lahey BB, Loeber R, Burke J, Rathouz PJ, McBurnett K. Waxing and waning in concert: Dynamic comorbidity of conduct disorder with other disruptive and emotional problems over 17 years among clinic-referred boys. *Journal of Abnormal Psychology.* 2002;111:556–567.

2. Lahey BB, Krueger RF, Rathouz PJ, Waldman ID, Zald DH. A hierarchical causal taxonomy of psychopathology across the life span. *Psychological Bulletin.* 2017;143:142–186.

3. Lahey BB, Rathouz PJ, Applegate B, et al. Testing structural models of DSM-IV symptoms of common forms of child and adolescent psychopathology. *Journal of Abnormal Child Psychology.* 2008;36:187–206.

4. Lahey BB, Applegate B, Waldman ID, Loft JD, Hankin BL, Rick J. The structure of child and adolescent psychopathology: Generating new hypotheses. *Journal of Abnormal Psychology.* 2004;113:358–385.

5. Willcutt EG, Nigg JT, Pennington BF, et al. Validity of DSM-IV attention deficit/hyperactivity disorder symptom dimensions and subtypes. *Journal of Abnormal Psychology.* 2012;121:991–1010.

6. Lahey BB, Lee SS, Sibley MH, Applegate B, Molina BSG, Pelham WE. Predictors of adolescent outcomes among 4–6-year-old children with attention-deficit/hyperactivity disorder. *Journal of Abnormal Psychology.* 2016;125(2):168–181.

7. Hechtman L, Swanson JM, Sibley MH, et al. Functional adult outcomes 16 years after childhood diagnosis of attention-deficit/hyperactivity disorder: MTA results. *Journal of the American Academy of Child and Adolescent Psychiatry.* 2016;55(11):945–952.

8. Owens EB, Zalecki C, Gillette P, Hinshaw SP. Girls with childhood ADHD as adults: Cross-domain outcomes by diagnostic persistence. *Journal of Consulting and Clinical Psychology.* 2017;85(7):723–736.

9. Sergeant JA. Modeling attention-deficit/hyperactivity disorder: A critical appraisal of the cognitive-energetic model. *Biological Psychiatry.* 2005;57:1248–1255.

10. Lahey BB, Pelham WE, Stein MA, et al. Validity of DSM-IV attention-deficit/hyperactivity disorder for younger children. *Journal of the American Academy of Child and Adolescent Psychiatry.* 1998;37:695–702.

11. Mak ADP, Chan AKW, Chan PKL, et al. Diagnostic outcomes of childhood ADHD in Chinese adults. *Journal of Attention Disorders.* 2020;24(1):126–135.

12. Stern A, Agnew-Blais JC, Danese A, et al. Associations between ADHD and emotional problems from childhood to young adulthood: A longitudinal genetically sensitive study. *Journal of Child Psychology and Psychiatry.* 2020;61(11):1234–1242.

13. Sun SH, Kuja-Halkola R, Faraone SV, et al. Association of psychiatric comorbidity with the risk of premature death among children and adults with attention-deficit/hyperactivity disorder. *JAMA Psychiatry.* 2019;76(11):1141–1149.

14. Chang Z, Quinn PD, Hur K, et al. Association between medication use for attention-deficit/hyperactivity disorder and risk of motor vehicle crashes. *JAMA Psychiatry.* 2017;74(6):597–603.

15. Roy A, Hechtman L, Arnold LE, et al. Childhood predictors of adult functional outcomes in the Multimodal Treatment Study of Attention-Deficit/Hyperactivity Disorder (MTA). *Journal of the American Academy of Child and Adolescent Psychiatry.* 2017;56(8):687–695.

16. Uchida M, Spencer TJ, Faraone SV, Biederman J. Adult outcome of ADHD: An overview of results from the MGH longitudinal family studies of pediatrically and psychiatrically referred youth with and without ADHD of both sexes. *Journal of Attention Disorders.* 2018;22(6):523–534.

17. Voigt RG, Katusic SK, Colligan RC, Killian JM, Weaver AL, Barbaresi WJ. Academic achievement in adults with a history of childhood attention-deficit/hyperactivity disorder: A population-based prospective study. *Journal of Developmental and Behavioral Pediatrics.* 2017;38(1):1–11.

18. Beauchaine TP, Ben-David I, Bos M. ADHD, financial distress, and suicide in adulthood: A population study. *Science Advances.* 2020;6(40):eaba1551.

19. Chronis-Tuscano A, Molina BSG, Pelham WE, et al. Very early predictors of adolescent depression and suicide attempts in children with attention-deficit/hyperactivity disorder. *Archives of General Psychiatry.* 2010;67:1044–1051.

20. Erskine HE, Norman RE, Ferrari AJ, et al. Long-term outcomes of attention-deficit/hyperactivity disorder and conduct disorder: A

systematic review and meta-analysis. *Journal of the American Academy of Child and Adolescent Psychiatry.* 2016;55(10):841–850.

21. Owens EB, Hinshaw SP. Childhood conduct problems and young adult outcomes among women with childhood attention-deficit/hyperactivity disorder (ADHD). *Journal of Abnormal Psychology.* 2016;125(2):220–232.

22. Meinzer MC, Pettit JW, Waxmonsky JG, Gnagy E, Molina BSG, Pelham WE. Does childhood attention-deficit/hyperactivity disorder (ADHD) predict levels of depressive symptoms during emerging adulthood? *Journal of Abnormal Child Psychology.* 2016;44(4):787–797.

23. Ilbegi S, Groenman AP, Schellekens A, et al. Substance use and nicotine dependence in persistent, remittent, and late-onset ADHD: A 10-year longitudinal study from childhood to young adulthood. *Journal of Neurodevelopmental Disorders.* 2018;10.

24. Molina BSG, Howard AL, Swanson JM, et al. Substance use through adolescence into early adulthood after childhood-diagnosed ADHD: Findings from the MTA longitudinal study. *Journal of Child Psychology and Psychiatry.* 2018;59(6):692–702.

25. Lahey BB, Class QA, Zald DH, Rathouz PJ, Applegate B, Waldman ID. Prospective test of the developmental propensity model of antisocial behavior: From childhood and adolescence into early adulthood. *Journal of Child Psychology and Psychiatry.* 2018;59(6):676–683.

26. Loeber R, Burke JD, Lahey BB, Winters A, Zera M. Oppositional defiant and conduct disorder: A review of the past 10 years, Part I. *Journal of the American Academy of Child and Adolescent Psychiatry.* 2000;39(12):1468–1484.

27. Burke JD, Rowe R, Boylan K. Functional outcomes of child and adolescent oppositional defiant disorder symptoms in young adult men. *Journal of Child Psychology and Psychiatry.* 2014;55(3):264–272.

28. Burke JD, Waldman I, Lahey BB. Predictive validity of childhood oppositional defiant disorder and conduct disorder: Implications for the DSM-V. *Journal of Abnormal Psychology.* 2010;119(4):739–751.

29. Evans SC, Pederson CA, Fite PJ, Blossom JB, Cooley JL. Teacher-reported irritable and defiant dimensions of oppositional defiant disorder: Social, behavioral, and academic correlates. *School Mental Health.* 2016;8(2):292–304.

30. Burt SA. Do etiological influences on aggression overlap with those on rule breaking? A meta-analysis. *Psychological Medicine.* 2013; 43:1801–1812.

31. Gordon RA, Lahey BB, Kawai E, Loeber R, Stouthamer-Loeber M, Farrington DP. Antisocial behavior and youth gang membership: Selection and socialization. *Criminology.* 2004;42(1):55–87.

32. Hare RD. *Without conscience: The disturbing world of the psychopaths among us.* New York, NY: Guilford; 1993.

33. Cleckley H. *The mask of sanity.* St. Louis, MO: Mosby; 1976.

34. Patrick CJ, Fowles DC, Krueger RF. Triarchic conceptualization of psychopathy: Developmental origins of disinhibition, boldness, and meanness. *Development and Psychopathology.* 2009;21:913–938.

35. Baskin-Sommers AR, Curtin JJ, Newman JP. Emotion-modulated startle in psychopathy: Clarifying familiar effects. *Journal of Abnormal Psychology.* 2013;122(2):458–468.

36. Hamilton RKB, Racer KH, Newman JP. Impaired integration in psychopathy: A unified theory of psychopathic dysfunction. *Psychological Review.* 2015;122(4):770–791.

37. Farrington DP. Antisocial personality from childhood to adulthood. *The Psychologist.* 1991;4:389–394.

38. Loeber R, Burke JD, Lahey BB. What are adolescent antecedents to antisocial personality disorder? *Criminal Behaviour and Mental Health.* 2002;12:24–26.

39. Fox B, DeLisi M. Psychopathic killers: A meta-analytic review of the psychopathy–homicide nexus. *Aggression and Violent Behavior.* 2019;44:67–79.

40. Hart SD, Hare RD. Psychopathy: Assessment and association with criminal conduct. In: Stoff DM, Breiling J, Maser JD, eds. *Handbook of antisocial behavior.* New York, NY: Wiley; 1997:22–35.

41. Loeber R, Keenan K, Lahey BB, Green SM, Thomas C. Evidence for developmentally based diagnoses of oppositional defiant disorder and conduct disorder. *Journal of Abnormal Child Psychology.* 1993;21(4):377–410.

42. Goldstein RB, Grant BF, Huang BJ, et al. Lack of remorse in antisocial personality disorder: Sociodemographic correlates, symptomatic presentation, and comorbidity with Axis I and Axis II disorders in the National Epidemiologic Survey on Alcohol and Related Conditions. *Comprehensive Psychiatry.* 2006;47(4):291–299.

43. Black DW. The natural history of antisocial personality disorder. *Canadian Journal of Psychiatry.* 2015;60(7):309–314.

44. Lahey BB, Class QA, Zald DH, Rathouz PJ, Applegate B, Waldman ID. Prospective test of the developmental propensity model of antisocial behavior: From childhood and adolescence into early adulthood. *Journal of Child Psychology and Psychiatry.* 2018;59:676–683.

45. Stenbacka M, Moberg T, Romelsjo A, Jokinen J. Mortality and causes of death among violent offenders and victims: A Swedish population based longitudinal study. *BMC Public Health.* 2012;12:38.

46. Shepherd JP, Shepherd I, Newcombe RG, Farrington D. Impact of antisocial lifestyle on health: Chronic disability and death by middle age. *Journal of Public Health.* 2009;31(4):506–511.

47. Krasnova A, Eaton WW, Samuels JF. Antisocial personality and risks of cause-specific mortality: Results from the Epidemiologic Catchment Area study with 27 years of follow-up. *Social Psychiatry and Psychiatric Epidemiology.* 2019;54(5):617–625.

48. Lahey BB, Loeber R, Burke JD, Applegate B. Predicting future antisocial personality disorder in males from a clinical assessment in childhood. *Journal of Consulting and Clinical Psychology.* 2005;73:389–399.

49. Rivenbark JG, Odgers CL, Caspi A, et al. The high societal costs of childhood conduct problems: Evidence from administrative records up to age 38 in a longitudinal birth cohort. *Journal of Child Psychology and Psychiatry.* 2018;59(6):703–710.

50. Robins LN. Conduct disorder. *Journal of Child Psychology and Psychiatry.* 1991;32:193–212.

51. Warren JI, Burnette M. Factor invariance of Cluster B psychopathology among male and female inmates and association with impulsive and violent behavior. *Journal of Forensic Psychiatry & Psychology.* 2012;23(1):40–60.

52. Lootens CM, Robertson CD, Mitchell JT, Kimbrel NA, Hundt NE, Nelson-Gray RO. Factors of impulsivity and Cluster B personality dimensions. *Journal of Individual Differences.* 2017;38(4):203–210.

53. Boudreaux MJ, South SC, Oltmanns TF. Symptom-level analysis of DSM-IV/DSM-5 personality pathology in later life: Hierarchical structure and predictive validity across self- and informant ratings. *Journal of Abnormal Psychology.* 2019;128(5):365–384.

54. Markon KE. Modeling psychopathology structure: A symptom-level analysis of Axis I and II disorders. *Psychological Medicine.* 2010;40:273–288.

55. Abel KM, Drake R, Goldstein JM. Sex differences in schizophrenia. *International Review of Psychiatry.* 2010;22(5):417–428.

56. Fischer B, Imtiaz S, Rudzinski K, Rehm J. Crude estimates of cannabis-attributable mortality and morbidity in Canada: Implications for public health focused intervention priorities. *Journal of Public Health.* 2016;38(1):183–188.

57. Hasin DS, Stinson FS, Ogburn E, Grant BF. Prevalence, correlates, disability, and comorbidity of DSM-IV alcohol abuse and dependence in the United States—Results from the National Epidemiologic Survey on Alcohol and Related Conditions. *Archives of General Psychiatry.* 2007;64(7):830–842.

58. Compton WM, Thomas YF, Stinson FS, Grant BF. Prevalence, correlates, disability, and comorbidity of DSM-IV drug abuse and dependence in the United States—Results from the National Epidemiologic Survey on Alcohol and Related Conditions. *Archives of General Psychiatry.* 2007;64(5):566–576.

59. Fridell M, Hesse M, Johnson E. High prognostic specificity of antisocial personality disorder in patients with drug dependence: Results from a five-year follow-up. *American Journal on Addictions.* 2006;15(3):227–232.

60. Buckner JD, Heimberg RG, Schneier FR, Liu SM, Wang S, Blanco C. The relationship between cannabis use disorders and social anxiety disorder

in the National Epidemiological Study of Alcohol and Related Conditions (NESARC). *Drug and Alcohol Dependence*. 2012;124(1–2):128–134.

61. Rioux C, Castellanos-Ryan N, Parent S, Vitaro F, Tremblay RE, Seguin JR. Age of cannabis use onset and adult drug abuse symptoms: A prospective study of common risk factors and indirect effects. *Canadian Journal of Psychiatry*. 2018;63(7):457–464.

62. Edwards G, Gross MM. Alcohol dependence: Provisional description of a clinical syndrome. *British Medical Journal*. 1976;1(6017):1058–1061.

63. Dierker L, Swendsen J, Rose J, He JP, Merikangas K; Tobacco Etiology Research Network. Transitions to regular smoking and nicotine dependence in the Adolescent National Comorbidity Survey (NCS-A). *Annals of Behavioral Medicine*. 2012;43(3):394–401.

64. Lopez-Quintero C, de los Cobos JP, Hasin DS, et al. Probability and predictors of transition from first use to dependence on nicotine, alcohol, cannabis, and cocaine: Results of the National Epidemiologic Survey on Alcohol and Related Conditions (NESARC). *Drug and Alcohol Dependence*. 2011;115(1–2):120–130.

65. Forman-Hoffman VL, Glasheen C, Batts KR. Marijuana use, recent marijuana initiation, and progression to marijuana use disorder among young male and female adolescents aged 12–14 living in US households. *Substance Abuse-Research and Treatment*. 2017;11:1–14.

66. Chandra M, Anthony JC. Cocaine dependence: "Side effects" and syndrome formation within 1–12 months after first cocaine use. *Drug and Alcohol Dependence*. 2020;206:107717.

67. Rivera OJS, Havens JR, Parker MA, Anthony JC. Risk of heroin dependence in newly incident heroin users. *JAMA Psychiatry*. 2018;75(8):863–864.

68. Bluthenthal RN, Simpson K, Ceasar RC, Zhao J, Wenger L, Kral AH. Opioid withdrawal symptoms, frequency, and pain characteristics as correlates of health risk among people who inject drugs. *Drug and Alcohol Dependence*. 2020;211:107932.

69. Hartley S, Simon N, Larabi A, et al. Effect of smoked cannabis on vigilance and accident risk using simulated driving in occasional and chronic users and the pharmacokinetic–pharmacodynamic relationship. *Clinical Chemistry*. 2019;65(5):684–693.

70. Martin JL, Gadegbeku B, Wu D, Viallon V, Laumon B. Cannabis, alcohol and fatal road accidents. *PLoS One*. 2017;12(11):e0187320.

71. Cerda M, Wall M, Keyes KM, Galea S, Hasin D. Medical marijuana laws in 50 states: Investigating the relationship between state legalization of medical marijuana and marijuana use, abuse and dependence. *Drug and Alcohol Dependence*. 2012;120(1–3):22–27.

72. Davenport S. Falling rates of marijuana dependence among heavy users. *Drug and Alcohol Dependence*. 2018;191:52–55.

73. Smart R, Pacula RL. Early evidence of the impact of cannabis legalization on cannabis use, cannabis use disorder, and the use of other

substances: Findings from state policy evaluations. *American Journal of Drug and Alcohol Abuse*. 2019;45(6):644–663.

74. Arterberry BJ, Padovano HT, Foster KT, Zucker RA, Hicks BM. Higher average potency across the United States is associated with progression to first cannabis use disorder symptom. *Drug and Alcohol Dependence*. 2019;195:186–192.

75. El Marroun H, Bolhuis K, Franken IHA, et al. Preconception and prenatal cannabis use and the risk of behavioural and emotional problems in the offspring: A multi-informant prospective longitudinal study. *International Journal of Epidemiology*. 2019;48(1):287–296.

76. El Marroun H, Tiemeier H, Franken IHA, et al. Prenatal cannabis and tobacco exposure in relation to brain morphology: A prospective neuroimaging study in young children. *Biological Psychiatry*. 2016;79(12):971–979.

77. Hasan A, von Keller R, Friemel CM, et al. Cannabis use and psychosis: A review of reviews. *European Archives of Psychiatry and Clinical Neuroscience*. 2020;270(4):403–412.

78. Arseneault L, Cannon M, Poulton R, Murray R, Caspi A, Moffitt TE. Cannabis use in adolescence and risk for adult psychosis: Longitudinal prospective study. *British Medical Journal*. 2002;325(7374):1212–1213.

5

Dimensions of Psychotic and Other Problems of Thought and Affect

The term *psychotic* refers to beliefs and experiences that essentially all members of a society consider to be baseless or false. Many of the broad range of problems described in this chapter involve psychotic beliefs, perceptual experiences, and other cognitive disturbances that can be said to put the person "out of touch with reality." In addition, they often involve emotions and atypical energy levels that can be markedly inconsistent with the situation. Cognition, emotion, and energy levels that are not consistent with reality can take a very serious toll on us, but recent research strongly suggests that each of these problems lies on a continuum and can be viewed in dimensional terms. Many persons experience relatively mild and short-lasting problems of these sorts that are not impairing in the long term.[1-3] Consulting with a psychologist or psychiatrist if you experience the problems described in this chapter is recommended, but be careful to accurately describe what you experience, how often it occurs, and whether it distresses you or interferes with your life. You do not want a psychiatrist to overreact and prescribe anti-psychotic medication if you do not need it. On the other hand, consultation with a professional should help you decide if you do or do not need help.

Not all of the dimensions described in this chapter involve what are usually considered to be psychotic problems, but recent research suggests that these several dimensions of psychological problems are more related than previously thought.[4,5] The dimensions described in this chapter are shown on the right-hand side of Figure 5.1, which is a repeat of the figure depicting the hierarchical structure of psychological problems that was presented in Chapter 2. When the dimensions of problems described here are distressing and impairing, a variety of categorical diagnoses are used in the *Diagnostic and Statistical Manual of Mental Disorders* (DSM). These diagnoses, which include dissociative

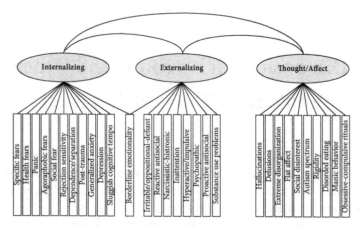

Figure 5.1 Hypothesized second-order internalizing, externalizing, and psychotic thought/affect dimensions of psychological problems.

disorder, schizophrenia, bipolar disorder, obsessive–compulsive disorder, and eating disorders, are traditionally not considered to be related. I suggest some potentially important ways in which they share important features as the chapter progresses, but much remains to be learned in further research.

Dissociative Problems

The two dimensions of dissociation problems described in this section involve altered perceptions of oneself and one's world, sometimes occurring together. They involve experiences that can be unnerving but usually are only problematic when they are repeated and persistent. Although these problems involve clear alterations of reality, they traditionally have not been considered to be true psychotic problems.

Depersonalization

Persons who are extreme on this dimension of psychological problems experience unrealistic perceptions of *themselves*. They may feel that their head is stuffed full of cotton or may experience tingling or light-headedness. They may feel they are numb and have no real emotions, and they sometimes feel detached from their own thoughts or feelings. They may feel that their body parts are enlarged or shrunken or not connected with the rest of their body. Some persons have so-called out of body experiences, feeling as if they are outside their own body, looking at themselves as an outside observer. Some persons experience time as being speeded up or slowed down. They may have difficulty recalling their own personal experiences. In some cases, they may feel that they are not actually real persons but are automatons with no control over their own actions. Indeed, they may be preoccupied with the question of whether they actually exist.

Derealization

This dimension is characterized by an unrealistic perception of one's *environment* rather than one's self. Some persons feel as if they are divided from their surroundings by something like a glass wall or a veil. They may perceive other people or their physical surroundings as unreal, unfamiliar, artificial, or distorted. They may view their surroundings as colorless, foggy, or lifeless. The outside world may seem either closer or farther away than usual, and sounds may be experienced as either softer or louder than usual.

Psychotic Problems

The problems described in this section capture a broad range of psychotic beliefs and perceptual experiences that are often markedly "out of touch with reality." There has long been evidence that psychotic problems can be thought of as being on a continuum.[6,7] At one end of the continuum, many individuals have psychotic experiences that are very mild, not distressing or impairing, transient, and are not signs that more serious problems will develop in the future.[8] For example, 11% of persons in Sweden and one-third of persons in the United States answered "yes" to questions such as the following: "Have you ever seen something that wasn't there that other people could not see?" and "Have you ever heard any voices that other people said did not exist?" Affirmative answers to such questions could represent naïve misunderstandings of what was being asked, but many studies suggest that genuine psychotic-like perceptual experiences such as these are more common in the general population than once believed.[9] Only a small proportion of persons who have these experiences will ever have problems serious enough to meet DSM diagnostic criteria for a psychotic disorder such as schizophrenia, however.[10]

When psychotic experiences are extreme and recurrent, most persons are impaired by them.[9,11-13] These problems are considered in DSM to define several different categorical diagnoses, including schizotypal personality disorder and schizophrenia. I make no distinction here between schizotypal personality disorder and schizophrenia because they appear to represent varying degrees of the same dimension of psychotic experiences.[14] This view is consistent with findings that the diagnosis of schizotypal personality disorder is often *prodromal* to the diagnosis of schizophrenia. This means that schizotypal problems emerge earlier and often, but certainly not always, predict the later diagnosis of schizophrenia. A study of the medical records of the entire Danish population found that 16% of young adults who met diagnostic criteria for schizotypal personality disorder met criteria for schizophrenia within the next 2 years and 33% met criteria for schizophrenia within 20 years.[15]

Hallucinations, Delusions, and Disorganization

I distinguish among a number of different but correlated dimensions of psychological problems that are used in DSM diagnoses. Here, I describe the several dimensions of psychological problems that are considered in DSM to be "positive symptoms" of schizotypal personality disorder, schizophrenia, and other forms of psychosis. They are not positive in the sense of being good but in the sense that they represent the *presence* of problems rather than the *absence* of adaptive characteristics, which DSM refers to as "negative symptoms" of psychosis. This distinction will become clearer as I describe these problems.

Hallucinations

The dimension of hallucinatory experiences is defined by sensory experiences that are inconsistent with reality in the sense of not being confirmed by others, such as hearing sounds, whispering, murmuring, or spoken voices that other people do not hear. This can sometimes include voices that command the person to do things. At times, persons experience other sensory experiences—seeing, smelling, or skin sensations—that are not confirmed by others.

Odd Beliefs and Delusions

This dimension of problems is defined by beliefs that nearly all members of society consider to be strange and false. Therefore, the culture or subculture in which the individual lives must be carefully considered, as cultures differ in the beliefs they consider to be false. The most common odd beliefs and delusions include the following: Some persons believe in clairvoyance—knowing things through extrasensory perception—or think they can read other people's minds through telepathy. Some individuals believe that other people can easily read *their* minds or may believe that their thoughts are being broadcast out loud and everyone can hear them. Persons who are extreme on this dimension may hold *delusions of influence*, such as the belief that someone has inserted or removed thoughts from their mind or that their mind is being controlled by other people—such as by people in another country for in a civilization in outer space. They may hold *ideas of reference*, which are beliefs that unrelated things in the world are referring to them directly, such as believing that the lyrics of a popular song were written only to send a message specifically to them or that cell phones were invented solely to send messages to them.

Paranoid delusions involve extreme suspiciousness and lack of trust in others based on the unjustified belief that others are trying to exploit, harm, or deceive them. Persons with extreme paranoid delusions are very uncomfortable in the presence of others, not because of social anxiety but, rather, because of their paranoid suspicions and beliefs about the harmful intentions of others. Social relationships take a serious toll when persons are on high alert that others will take advantage of them; are suspicious of the intensions of their spouses, bosses, and fellow employees; and are preoccupied with worries that their friends are disloyal. Persons who experience paranoid delusions are reluctant to confide in others for fear the information will be used to harm them, and they often read demeaning or threatening hidden messages into benign remarks. They may believe without justification that their character or reputation is being attacked and react angrily with unjustified counterattacks. They often hold extreme grudges and are unforgiving of others.

Somatic delusions are obviously false beliefs that the person has a physical illness or disability, including improbable illnesses such as brain rot caused by an unknown kind of cosmic radiation. *Grandiose beliefs* are exaggerated positive beliefs about oneself that other people think are false, such as an extreme sense of self-importance, believing they have almost magical talents and powers, being convinced that they are on an improbable mission such as saving the country or the world, or being preoccupied with their unrealistic and unlikely plans to achieve extreme success. These grandiose beliefs may be religious delusions, such as that one is a spiritual savior, has a unique relationship with the gods, or is possessed by a devil. In some cases, individual experience an *erotomanic delusion*, which is the baseless belief that someone, usually a famous person they have never met, is in love with them. In rare instances, persons hold the delusional belief that they are possessed by multiple personalities.

Disorganized Thinking and Speech

Some persons exhibit disorganized thinking and speech, which is viewed as another positive "symptom" of schizophrenia in DSM when extreme. The person's thoughts may seem to have become derailed, loosely connected, or incoherent. Their speech and writing may appear to be very odd and difficult to understand because their thoughts are vague, loosely connected by little apparent logic, or the writing is extremely stereotyped, highly metaphorical, or overly elaborate. *Hebephrenic behavior* refers to an extreme form of disorganized behavior characterized by unpredictable changes from emotional flatness to high levels of excitement and agitation that sometimes includes a maladaptive form of extreme silliness, such as throwing feces at people. In some instances, persons experience the opposite of disorganized and agitated movement; *catatonic behavior* is defined by an extreme lack of motor movement, an absence of speech (mutism), and at times an almost motionless state of apparent stupor.

Outcomes of Psychotic Problems

There is substantial variability in the long-term outcomes for persons whose psychotic behaviors meet DSM binary diagnostic criteria for schizophrenia. One 34-year-long study followed 128 persons who were given the diagnosis of schizophrenia and whose problems were serious enough to receive inpatient treatment in mental hospitals. Almost 10% of these persons could be said to have completely improved and maintained that recovery for many years, and another 10% improved substantially. Nonetheless, schizophrenic problems persisted in the remaining 80% of diagnosed persons. Some of these individual showed a high level of relatively constant psychotic problems, but most fluctuated irregularly in their functioning over their lifetimes, sometimes being relatively free of schizophrenic problems for a year or longer but then returning to impaired psychotic functioning.[16]

Schizoid Problems

People are said to behave in schizoid ways when they display an apparent absence of the feelings and actions that link people to one another. *Social disinterest* and *detachment* are central features of the DSM diagnosis of schizoid personality disorder. At the extreme of this dimension, individuals appear to lack any interest in having social relationships. They exhibit social detachment by having no close friends, no sexual relationships, and sparse interaction with family members. They usually or always choose to engage in solitary activities. They often display an emotional coldness toward others and seem to be indifferent to praise or criticism from others. *Impoverished speech* is common in persons with other schizoid characteristics. People differ along a continuum of how much they communicate with others, but at the extreme of this dimension, the individual speaks infrequently and communicates very little information when speaking. Some individuals also exhibit levels of *impoverished volition*, meaning they engage in little voluntary action, including taking care of adequate hygiene.

Flat affect and *anhedonia* refer to an apparent blunting or flattening of emotions, revealed by the person showing little proportional positive or negative emotional response to either favorable or tragic events. Being told that a parent has died may evoke little sadness, just as being told that they had inherited millions from a distant relative would be greeted with little pleasure or excitement. They express their emotions in restricted and shallow ways that do not appear to reveal any genuine feelings. Individuals with such problems get bored easily, appear to experience diminished pleasure, and do not seek or participate in what most people consider to be enjoyable activities. As noted in Chapter 3, such anhedonia also is often part of the dimension of depression. In addition, persons who are high on the psychopathic/proactive antisocial behavior dimension also are easily bored and express their emotions in shallow ways. Again, the field does not yet know how to deal with such psychological problems that are part of multiple dimensions.

Although the *schiz-* root of the term *schizoid* is the same as that in schizotypal personality disorder and schizophrenia, there are complicated similarities and difference between schizoid behavior and those other dimensions of problems. Note that schizoid behavior does not include psychotic beliefs or perceptions such as those that are part of schizotypal and schizophrenic behavior. Persons with these problems are in touch with reality, but they have little interest in social relationships and polite conventions.

The next statement that I make may be a bit confusing at first. When schizoid problems *co-occur* with the "positive symptoms" of hallucinations, delusions, and disorganized behavior and language, they are considered to be "negative symptoms" of schizophrenia. As noted previously, lack of social interest, diminished pleasure, emotional flatness, impoverished speech, and lack of volition are referred to as negative in this context because they are viewed as the *absence* of adaptive social and emotional behavior. For example, emotional flatness and anhedonia are referred to as negative symptoms of schizophrenia because they involves the absence of adaptive positive affect and motivation.

In contrast, when schizoid problems occur on their own—that is, in the absence of hallucinations, delusions, and disorganized behavior and language and other positive symptoms of schizophrenia—they are considered to be the symptoms of the categorical diagnosis of schizoid personality disorder in the DSM. Schizoid problems by themselves do not appear to be a precursor to the diagnosis of schizophrenia.[15] That is, persons with even serious schizoid problems without schizotypal odd beliefs and related problems rarely progress to a diagnosis of schizophrenia.

Manic Problems

The problems that define this dimension of psychological problems are viewed as the symptoms of the binary diagnosis of manic episodes in the DSM. When high levels of these problems alternate in some way with episodes of depression, they are part of the broader diagnostic category of *bipolar disorder*, although under some conditions the diagnosis of bipolar disorder is given to persons who display only high levels of manic behavior. Mania is quite reasonably considered to be a problem of mood, but note that the beliefs and perceptions of persons whose behavior is described as manic can be unrealistic enough to put them "out of touch with reality" and in conflict with others.

Manic behavior represents a *marked change* from the person's usual mood and behavior that generally only lasts a matter of weeks or months, although the episodes often recur and sometimes recur multiple times. Often, the individual returns to typical patterns of behavior following manic episodes, but most persons who experience extreme episodes of manic behavior will experience episodes of depression during some part of the time between manic episodes. Only a minority of persons who experience high levels of depression will also experience episodes of mania, but most persons who experience manic episodes will eventually experience depressive episodes.

The change in the person's mood varies from individual to individual. Often, the change is to an unrealistically elated state, involving elevated self-esteem, positive mood, and high levels of energy. These seemingly positive changes can be extreme enough to interfere in important ways with life functioning. For these persons, the experience of life during a manic episode is the opposite of episodes of depression, in which persons are deeply sad, lethargic, slow moving, uninterested in pleasure, and unrealistically pessimistic and hopeless.[17] For many other individuals who exhibit high levels of manic problems, however, the change in mood is to higher than usual irritability rather than to euphoric happiness.

Regardless of the nature of the mood change, persons who are extreme on the mania dimension can be filled with energy, optimistic in grandiose ways, and enthusiastic about seeking pleasure and pursuing lofty goals. Their self-esteem is often markedly elevated to unrealistic and grandiose levels. They are more talkative than usual and often exhibit "pressured speech," in which it seems as if they have to keep talking. Some persons experience a rapid flight of ideas in which their thoughts seem to be racing in their heads, and they are often more distractible than usual. Individuals who are extreme on the manic dimension often have a decreased need for sleep, waking up feeling rested after only a few hours of sleep. It is common for them to focus on themselves and disregard family obligations and other responsibilities. They often experience an increase in sexual interest and activity, often having sex with persons outside of their established relationship. It is also common for them to show an increase in unrealistic goal-directed activities that have the potential for disastrous financial consequences (e.g., unrestrained buying sprees, foolish business investments, or quitting one's job to pursue unrealistic goals).

Even when elation is the predominant mood change, irritability can be a problem. When relatives and other people try to reason with elated persons to stop their risky and unwise behavior, they are often met with extreme irritability and anger. This makes irritability a common part of manic behavior because the unrealistic goals and behavior are often met with frequent opposition from others.

Obsessive–Compulsive Problems

Obsessive–Compulsive Rituals

Obsessive–compulsive rituals are not usually viewed as being related to psychotic behavior even though they clearly reflect a kind of loss of contact reality.[5] Some individuals experience recurrent and unwelcome thoughts or feelings that others believe are unrealistic. These thoughts and feelings create anxiety, disgust, or other negative emotions and are therefore very difficult for the person to ignore or suppress. Such upsetting *obsessions* are often reduced or eliminated by repetitive thoughts or behaviors that are performed in a rigid or stereotype manner, referred to as *compulsions*. The obsessive concerns and their compulsive remedies often seem unreasonable to others, but they must be distressing to the individual or must interfere with their life functioning to be considered a psychological problem. This is often the case because the rituals take up a lot of productive time or they are odd enough to alienate other persons who observe them.

The specific problems experienced by persons who are high on the dimension of obsessive–compulsive rituals are varied. Some individuals experience repeated worry about something dangerous happening, such as an intruder entering the house because the doors are not locked or the home catching fire because the stove was not turned off. These anxiety-provoking thoughts are temporarily reduced by frequently checking door locks and stoves—but only temporarily. Such compulsive checking rituals are common in the population and not always impairing when minor, but they can become distressing, time-consuming, and interfere with life functioning.

Maladaptive obsessions can include repeated feelings of being contaminated by filth or germs when there is no evidence of actual contamination. These experiences elicit anxiety or disgust, which is relieved by compulsive washing or cleaning. Obsessive–compulsive washing rituals can become time-consuming and can cause skin damage due to frequent washing. Some individuals are obsessively concerned that the things in their environments are not sufficiently ordered or symmetrical, which leads to irrational anxiety that is relieved temporarily by compulsively arranging or ordering those things. Some persons obsessively count the things in their environments or feel that they have to repeat actions a certain number of times to avoid some kind of calamity. Individuals may feel that taboo thoughts repeatedly come into their heads or may experience intrusive and compelling urges to yell obscenities or do other inappropriate things. These urges may be controlled with compulsive prayer or religious rituals.

Traditionally, obsessive–compulsive rituals have been thought of as part of the internalizing domain because anxiety is often experienced when the person attempts to deny the obsession or not engage in the compulsive remedy; however, more recent evidence suggests that these rituals could be more strongly related to the domain of thought and affect problems.[4,5] This issue is unresolved because of the lack of sufficient studies on this topic.

Compulsive Rigidity and Perfectionism

The problems of rigidity that I describe here have traditionally been considered to be symptoms of the two binary diagnoses of obsessive–compulsive disorder and autistic spectrum disorders, and they may play a role in anorexic eating disorders defined later. Rigidity and perfectionism do not always cause problems for people, but they often do, with the impairment ranging from mild to serious.

Compulsive rigidity is defined by a pattern of behavior that can be desirable in moderation but becomes a problem when it is inflexible and extreme. A cardinal feature of this dimension is a generally rigid and inflexible approach to activities and tasks, including a preoccupation with rules, details, and organization to the point that it interferes with the purpose of the activity. Persons who are extreme on this dimension also often have very high and rigid moral standards. They often demonstrate a high level of devotion to work, but sometimes they are so exacting and perfectionistic in their expectations for the behavior of themselves and others that it interferes with both relationships and tasks. Some individuals rigidly hoard money and spend it on both themselves and others in a miserly manner that goes beyond the necessity of their resources.

Autistic Spectrum Problems

The defining issue of autism spectrum problems is difficulties in social interactions, but I begin by describing the problems of rigid and repetitive behavior to draw attention to their similarity to compulsive problems of rigidity.

Autistic Rigidity and Repetitive Behavior

The behaviors described here are considered to be symptoms of the categorical diagnosis of autism spectrum disorder when they are extreme enough to cause distress or interfere with social relationships and other aspects of adaptive functioning. Some individuals engage frequently in repetitive and stereotyped motor movements, such as rocking their body, spinning objects, or other stereotyped movements of objects. They often repeat other ritualized behaviors as well, such as stereotyped greetings. They may rigidly repeat back statements that are said to them rather than generating their own speech, which is known as *echolalia*, or they may repeat idiosyncratic phrases. Individuals who are extreme on this dimension may be inflexibly insistent on "sameness," with even small changes in routines or the environment causing them distress. This may include insistently eating the same foods every day, needing to always take the same route when walking, and difficulties making transitions from one activity or situation to a new one. They often have narrowly circumscribed interests, such as a fascination with subway schedules, that are intense and perseverative. Atypical responses to sensations are common in persons with other autistic problems, including excessive touching or smelling of certain objects or a fascination with lights or movement and atypical negative reactions to certain sounds or textures that are not aversive to most persons but sometimes involve an apparent insensitivity to pain or extremes of temperature.

Autistic Spectrum Social Problems

Although rigid behavior is an important component of autistic problem, the defining issue of the autism spectrum is mild to severe difficulties in social interactions. Autism spectrum problems always begin in early childhood, but not everyone with social relationship problems that start in childhood should be viewed as being on the autism spectrum, of course. Recall from Chapter 2 that there are many reasons for social relationship problems. Autism spectrum problems are found in persons with a broad range of levels of intelligence, but many individuals with serious autistic-like problems have intelligence scores that are well below average. It is important, therefore, to use the term autism spectrum only if the problems are more unusual and impairing than expected for the person's intellectual level.

Like persons who are said to exhibit schizoid behavior, some persons with autistic-like problems prefer to be alone and are not interested in social relationships. Others want friendships but behave in ways that interfere with them. These problems in social behavior include an inflexible and demanding self-centered focus on their own interests and difficulties sharing the interests of other people. Persons extreme on this dimension often display a lack of typical reciprocal verbal communication and have important problems interpreting the nonverbal behavior of others. Their own nonverbal behavior is also often atypical, such as a low level of appropriate eye contact with others, inappropriately invading the personal space of others, and often not responding when their name is called. Some persons on this spectrum seem indifferent to appropriate physical contact, and others find it to be aversive. In addition, they sometimes smile or laugh at inappropriate times during social interactions.

Anorexic and Bulimic Eating Problems

The dimensions defined in this section describe dangerous patterns of eating that often result in life-threatening malnutrition. Like many of the other dimensions of psychological problems described in this chapter, they are characterized by highly rigid behavior and distorted perceptions, but they are limited to issues of eating and body image.

Anorexic Eating Problems

This pattern of insufficient eating is associated with a higher level of mortality than any other dimension of psychological problems. It not only can lead to death due to emaciation and malnutrition sufficient to cause heart attacks or multiple organ failure but also is associated with an increased risk of suicide.[18] Persons with eating problems may perceive themselves to be overweight despite their being of normal weight or even severely underweight.[18] These distorted perceptions of their body weight, which have been referred to as *body image disturbance*, are not usually viewed as hallucinatory, but they certainly reflect a marked distortion of reality. Frequently, the false perception of being overweight causes a high level of distress that is sometimes unbearable for the individual and can be relieved only by severe undereating. This pattern of undereating is rigidly adhered to and often results in severely restricted caloric intake. Persons with these problems often weigh themselves frequently to monitor their weight and avoid weight gain. Very often, the individual with these problems keeps their rigidly restricted eating private from family members and roommates to avoid scrutiny and pressure from others to eat more. Sometimes, their low weight is also controlled by frequent exercise, the use of laxatives, and self-induced vomiting after eating.

Bulimic and Binge Eating Problems

Bulimia is defined by frequently recurring episodes of binge eating that go well beyond the point of satiety, in which very large amounts of food are eaten. Individuals with this problem often do not feel that they are in control of their binge eating and compensate for bingeing by inducing vomiting, using laxatives or diuretics to rid themselves of the food, and may engage in periods of fasting and excessive exercise to offset the large intake of calories. The repeated vomiting not only causes damage to the throat and teeth but also can result in dehydration and electrolyte imbalances that can cause heart attack or stroke. *Binge eating* is defined by frequent and uncontrolled eating beyond the point of satiety but not followed by purging, excessive exercise, or fasting. Understandably, it often results in being overweight or obese, although binge eating is certainly not the usual cause of obesity.

Conversion Somatic Problems

Some persons experience impairing somatic (bodily) difficulties for which there is no known medical basis. These resemble symptoms of neurological disorders to a considerable degree, but they do not correspond with any recognized neurological condition. This dimension of psychological problems includes muscle weakness, paralysis, tremors, problems swallowing, speech problems, seizures, anesthesia (lack of sensation), and sudden blindness or other sensory loss. Persons with conversion problems often display telltale signs of the absence of neurological dysfunction, however. For example, persons with paralysis of the legs are observed to move their legs normally when asleep, which does not occur in true paralysis due to neurological damage. Similarly, persons with conversion problems who have areas of numbness on the hands and other places do not have numbness in areas that correspond with nerve pathways. The term conversion somatic problems is used only for cases in which malingering—intentionally lying about medical symptoms to get out of work or for personal gain—is not suspected. Because conversion problems do not appear to be the result of a medical problem, they are typically viewed as "psychological" in origin, although what that means has never been specified satisfactorily. It is important to keep in mind that not detecting a known medical cause of these problems does not mean that there is not one. Medical diagnosis is not an exact science, and it is possible that future medical discoveries will paint some of these problems in a different light. These problems are placed at the end of the description of psychological problems partly because they have not been studied sufficiently to know how they are correlated with other psychological problems.

References

1. van Os J, Linscott RJ, Myin-Germeys I, Delespaul P, Krabbendam L. A systematic review and meta-analysis of the psychosis continuum: Evidence for a psychosis proneness–persistence–impairment model of psychotic disorder. *Psychological Medicine*. 2009;39(2):179–195.

2. Michal M, Wiltink J, Subic-Wrana C, et al. Prevalence, correlates, and predictors of depersonalization experiences in the German general population. *Journal of Nervous and Mental Disease*. 2009;197(7):499–506.

3. Aderibigbe YA, Bloch RR, Walker WR. Prevalence of depersonalization and derealization experiences in a rural population. *Social Psychiatry and Psychiatric Epidemiology*. 2001;36(2):63–69.

4. Caspi A, Houts RM, Belsky DW, et al. The p factor: One general psychopathology factor in the structure of psychiatric disorders? *Clinical Psychological Science*. 2014;2:119–137.

5. Caspi A, Moffitt TE. All for one and one for all: Mental disorders in one dimension. *American Journal of Psychiatry*. 2018;175(9):831–844.

6. Van Os J, Verdoux H, Bijl R, Ravelli A. Psychosis as an extreme of continuous variation in dimensions of psychopathology. In: Gattaz WF, Häfner H, eds. *Search for the causes of schizophrenia*. Vol. 4. New York: Springer; 1999:56–79.

7. Clark LA, Watson D, Reynolds S. Diagnosis and classification of psychopathology: Challenges to the current system and future directions. *Annual Review of Psychology*. 1995;46:121–153.

8. Wusten C, Schlier B, Jaya ES, et al. Psychotic experiences and related distress: A cross-national comparison and network analysis based on 7141 participants from 13 countries. *Schizophrenia Bulletin*. 2018;44(6):1185–1194.

9. Linscott RJ, van Os J. Systematic reviews of categorical versus continuum models in psychosis: Evidence for discontinuous subpopulations underlying a psychometric continuum. Implications for DSM-V, DSM-VI, and DSM-VII. Annual Review of Clinical Psychology. 6:391–419.

10. Legge SE, Jones HJ, Kendall KM, et al. Association of genetic liability to psychotic experiences with neuropsychotic disorders and traits. *JAMA Psychiatry*. 2019;76(12):1256–1265.

11. Linscott RJ, van Os J. An updated and conservative systematic review and meta-analysis of epidemiological evidence on psychotic experiences in children and adults: On the pathway from proneness to persistence to dimensional expression across mental disorders. *Psychological Medicine*. 2013;43(6):1133–1149.

12. McGrath JJ, Saha S, Al-Hamzawi A, et al. Psychotic experiences in the general population: A cross-national analysis based on 31,261 respondents from 18 countries. *JAMA Psychiatry*. 2015;72(7):697–705.

13. Laurens KR, Tzoumakis S, Dean K, Harris F, Carr VJ, Green MJ. Population profiles of child-reported psychotic-like experiences and their differential association with other psychopathologies. *British Journal of Clinical Psychology*. 2020;59(1):22–38.

14. Moussa-Tooks AB, Bailey AJ, Bolbecker AR, Viken RJ, O'Donnell BF, Hetrick WP. Bifactor structure of the Schizotypal Personality

Questionnaire across the schizotypy spectrum. *Journal of Personality Disorder.* 2020;34:466.

15. Hjorthoj C, Albert N, Nordentoft M. Association of substance use disorders with conversion from schizotypal disorder to schizophrenia. *JAMA Psychiatry.* 2018;75(7):733–739.

16. Newman SC, Bland RC, Thompson AH. Long-term course and outcome in schizophrenia: A 34-year follow-up study in Alberta, Canada. *Psychological Medicine.* 2012;42(10):2137–2143.

17. Alloy LB, Nusslock R. Future directions for understanding adolescent bipolar spectrum disorders: A reward hypersensitivity perspective. *Journal of Clinical Child and Adolescent Psychology.* 2019;48(4):669–683.

18. Engel MM, Keizer A. Body representation disturbances in visual perception and affordance perception persist in eating disorder patients after completing treatment. *Scientific Reports.* 2017;7.

6

Hierarchical Nature
of Psychological Problems

A dimensional approach makes it easier for us to see some important things about psychological problems that reveal their fundamental nature. As I have been saying, when researchers use dimensional measures of psychological problems in their studies, it is obvious that all dimensions of psychological problems are positively correlated with one another. That is, people with high scores on one dimension of psychological problem are more likely than chance to exhibit high levels of other dimensions of problems. Why is this important? Although each dimension of psychological problems has some unique characteristics, the fact that they are all correlated tells us that they also share some important things in common.

A central message of this book is that the correlations among dimensions of psychological problem are ubiquitous, but *these correlations are not uniform in magnitude*. By that, I simply mean that some pairs of dimensions of psychological problems are more strongly correlated than other pairs. This is highly important because these patterns of varying magnitudes of correlations among psychological reveal a *hierarchy of correlations* among psychological problems that can guide us as we try to discover the causes and mechanisms that are shared by all kinds of problems and the best ways to prevent and reduce psychological problems.

Bear with me while I draw a simple analogy to explain what I mean by a hierarchy of correlations. Suppose I show you a table covered by 45 different edible fruits, each with a name tag. At first, it looks like a disorganized scatter of fruit, including a couple you have never seen before. Having a curious scientific nature, you carefully look at their skins, smell them, and you cut them open to see and taste their flesh and look at their seeds. Furthermore, you decide to organize the fruit on the table to make better sense of what you are learning about the fruit. First, you notice that the 5 fruits with labels that say Red Delicious, Rome, Gala, Fuji, and Granny Smith share a lot of characteristics. Although they are each different in some ways, you group them together based on their similarities in skin, seeds, taste, and aroma. And being nobody's fool, you call this group of fruit apples. You similarly group another set of 5 fruits together into the category of oranges (the ones labeled Valencia, Seville, Mandarin, Navel, and Blood), another 5 fruits go into the category of pears (Anjou, Asian, Bartlett, Bosc, and Comice), and then you make similar groups of grapefruits, limes, quince, plums, apricots, and peaches. This organizes the 45 fruits into nine categories based on their similarities, so you have greatly reduced the disorganized complexity of what was put in front of you.

Then you notice that the apples have some features in common with the pears and quince. Despite their differences, they all have a thin skin, sweet grainy flesh, and multiple seeds. You decide that a *hierarchy* with both lower and higher order categories would help organize the fruit even more. So you group the apples, pears, and quince together in a second-order category (which you later learn that biologists call the genus *Cydonia*) both because they are all pretty similar to one another and because they differ in some ways from the other fruit. You put the oranges, limes, and grapefruit in a category that you call citrus on the basis of their leathery skins and flesh that is divided into sections, and you group the plums, apricots, and peaches (which biologists call genus *Prunus*) together because they are the only fruit on the table with a single pit instead of multiple seeds. Now you have organized all of the 45 fruits into the hierarchy illustrated in Figure 6.1 that initially groups the individual fruit into nine first-order categories, then groups those nine categories into just three second-order categories, and finally groups all of the fruit into a single category that you cleverly call *edible fruit*.

You have created a nifty hierarchical structure that helps you understand the fruits in an organized way by beginning with 45 individual elements and progressing from the bottom up into nine first-order categories, with those categories being organized into three second-order categories of edible fruit. You smile at your accomplishment and ask if you can have all of the 45 items on the table because you have worked up a bit of an appetite.

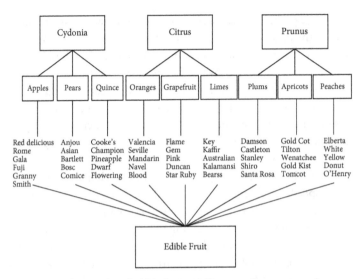

Figure 6.1 A hierarchy of edible fruits to illustrate the concept of hierarchical taxonomy.

Why did I take you through this exercise? Because we will now create a similar hierarchical classification of psychological problems using the same bottom-up approach based on similarities. Like the hierarchy of fruit, it will help us understand psychological problems by reducing the seeming complexity in them. The big difference is that this hierarchy will be based on empirically observed correlations among psychological problems.

Hierarchy of Psychological Problems

First- and Second-Order Dimensions of Psychological Problems

A number of studies of large numbers of children and adolescents— and a growing number of studies of adults—have measured a broad range of specific psychological problems. They found them all to be correlated with one another, albeit to varying degrees. For example, the specific problems that define depression—unhappiness, lack of interest in the pleasures of life, feelings of worthlessness, and the like—are highly correlated with one another, meaning that these specific problems often—but not invariably—co-occur in the same persons. Thus, if we count the number of these specific psychological problems (or sum ratings of the frequency and severity of each problem), we can consider the sum to *quantitatively measure* the dimension of depression. Many studies have similarly revealed many other such highly correlated dimensions of psychological problems.[1,2]

Thus, at the lowest level of the hierarchy of psychological problems, sets of specific problems are correlated enough—meaning that they co-occur enough—to treat them as members of the same dimensions. This is the equivalent to your seeing that Galas, Granny Smiths, and the others were similar enough to group together as apples. Critically, the studies of psychological problems have revealed that all of the dimensions of psychological problems are also correlated to varying extents in a clearly discernable pattern. For example, the dimensions of depression, fears, and worries are more highly correlated with one another than they are with other dimensions of psychological problems.[3–6] Thus, it is common for people to exhibit a mixture of problems that define the dimensions of depression, fears, and worries. Crucially, this is not what we would expect after reading the DSM, which implies that each person with significant psychological problems would exhibit only the "symptoms" of a *single* mental disorder. The reality is, however, that psychological problems do not occur in neat packets that fit the binary diagnostic criteria written in the DSM. Psychological problems color outside the lines. This fundamentally important fact is obscured by the Procrustean beds of the diagnostic categories used in the DSM that focus our attention on the symptoms of only a single diagnosis.

Similarly, the dimensions of psychological problems that have traditionally been considered to be "symptoms" of attention-deficit/hyperactivity disorder (ADHD), conduct problems, oppositional and defiant behavior, and substance use problems also are all correlated enough to define the different second-order externalizing dimension.[7–9] The important message here is that the patterns of correlations among specific psychological problems allow us to define dimensions and the pattern of correlations among dimensions allow us to define *second-order dimensions of psychological problems*.

Correlated Second-Order Dimensions of Psychological Problems

The patterns of correlations among psychological problems described previously have been well described since the 1960s.[10] This is another way in which the "revolutionary" thesis of this book is based on an *old* approach whose time had not yet come. For most of the time since the 1960s, psychologists and psychiatrists ignored an obvious and important fact about the pattern of corrections among psychopathological problems: Second-order internalizing and externalizing dimensions also are *positively correlated with one another*. Recent large studies conducted mostly with children and adolescents in the general population confirm that every internalizing dimension of psychological problems is positively correlated with every externalizing dimension at above chance levels, albeit to varying degrees.[3,5,9,11,12] All dimensions of psychological problems are correlated with one another, but that fact ran so counter to the belief fostered by the DSM that mental disorders are distinct and separate that the correlation was ignored! I agree with the many theorists[13–15] who now assert that these widespread correlations among every form of psychological problem are among the most important and potentially informative facts about the nature of psychological problems. I will try to explain why in the rest of this chapter.

General Factor of Psychological Problems

Again, one potentially informative way of thinking about the ubiquitous correlations among all dimensions of psychological problems is to posit that, to varying extents, all dimensions of psychological problems reflect something that is *common* to every sort of psychological problem. This is a revolutionary proposition that runs counter to the assumptions underlying the DSM, but to understand what I mean by it, we need to look back to the past again.

An important idea offered in 1904 by Charles Spearman[16] provides us with a useful way of thinking about psychological problems. Spearman was studying intelligence and he noticed that the many specific facets of intelligence (short-term memory, analogical reasoning, and the like) were all positively correlated. People are often higher on one facet than another, to be sure, but in general, people with strong ability in one area of intelligence are relatively strong in all areas. Spearman hypothesized that every specific mental ability was partly unique but also reflected a *general factor of intelligence,* which he called *g.* Using Spearman's *g* as an analogy, Ernest Jones suggested in an address to the British Psychoanalytic Society in 1946 that there may be a similar general factor of psychological problems that underlies all forms of psychological problems.[17] Jones speculated that the general factor that underlies all psychological problems is based on a general inability to regulate emotional reactions to frustration and psychological conflicts. I only recently learned about Jones' prescient hypothesis, but some ideas are so obvious that they keep occurring to people who look at the same data. In 2011 and 2012, I was part of a group that again had the idea that the ubiquitous correlations among categorical mental disorder in a large sample of adults may reflect a general factor of psychological problems. This time, however, we used a modern form of the statistical method Spearman had invented to study the general factor of psychological problems rather than offering a theory based on informal observations as Jones did. Our papers[4,18] were followed by an influential paper by Avshalon Caspi, Terrie Moffitt, and colleagues[12] that used similar statistical methods also to argue for a general factor of psychological problems, which they nicknamed p. Those first papers have been cited more than 1,500 times and have revived the discussion of a potential general factor of psychological problems that I am sorry Ernest Jones did not live to see.

Many subsequent studies of large samples have consistently shown that the hypothesized general factor of psychological problems must be taken seriously because it predicts many indicators of future distress and impaired functioning better than the specific dimensions of problems do. The general factor of psychological problems in childhood, adolescence, and adulthood is the strongest predictor of lack of success in the classroom,[19] reduced educational attainment,[20] poor work adjustment and financial difficulties,[20] use of outpatient and inpatient mental health services,[20,21] incarceration for crimes,[21] and suicide attempts and self-harm.[4,22]

In recent years, many other psychologists and psychiatrists have similarly argued that psychological problems are better viewed as a hierarchy of *correlated dimensions* than as distinct categorical diagnoses.[1,2,23–26] Their descriptions of psychological problems aim to be comprehensive, including both what were previously viewed in DSM-IV as "clinical disorders" and "personality disorders."[14] To fully evaluate these proposals, we will need to use comprehensive measures of all psychological problems in future studies that do not yet exist to reveal all of the first- and second-order dimensions in an empirical bottom-up fashion—starting with specific psychological problems and building up to higher order dimensions. When you looked at the fruit on the table, you had no idea how many second-order categories you would identify until you examined them. When you looked carefully, however, the patterns of similarities revealed the hierarchy. To be most informative, future studies of the dimensions of psychopathology need to be based on measures of the most comprehensive set of specific psychological problems possible and let the correlations in the data define the hierarchy dimensions. As shown in Figure 6.2, it is likely that the correlations among the various dimensions of psychological problems can be viewed as a hierarchy, with a general factor of psychopathology at the highest level of the hierarchy.*

To repeat, I am one of many scientists arguing that there is a hierarchy of correlations among dimensions of psychological problems.[2,23,25,27,28] As scientists often do, we do not agree on all the details about this hierachy,[29] but our views have far more commonalities than differences.

---

* Notice that the general factor is at the "highest" level of the hierarchy conceptually because it is defined by correlations among all of the dimensions, but it is portrayed at the bottom of Figure 6.2 to make it easier to render graphically

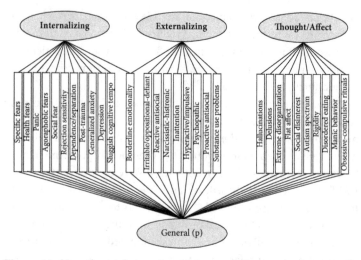

Figure 6.2 Hypothesized second-order internalizing, externalizing, and psychotic thought/affect dimensions of psychological problems, showing the hypothesized general factor of psychopathology (p).

Psychological Nature of the General Factor Hypothesis

So far, I have defined the general factor of psychopathology only in statistical terms—in terms of the patterns of correlations among dimensions. Now it is time to ask what the general factor of psychopathology represents in psychological terms? Can we say that all dimensions of psychopathology are correlated because they all reflect individual differences in some key psychological process (or processes) that increases risk for every dimension of psychopathology in a nonspecific way? The answer is that we do not know yet. Serious research on this question only began in 2011,[18] and we simply do not yet have enough information to be certain. Reminiscent of the insightful speculation of Ernest Jones in 1946, there is strong evidence that a general tendency to experience high levels of negative emotions—perhaps due to deficits in the mechanisms that regulate emotions—is associated with the general factor.[2,27,30] There also is less conclusive evidence that lower levels of cognitive abilities, including deficits in so-called executive functions, which regulate attention and impulsive behavior, may be related to the general factor of psychological problems.[2,29,31] There is far more to learn than we already know, but we can still make use of the general factor in understanding what processes are related to all dimensions of psychological problems.

Causal Hierarchy Hypothesis

We are making progress toward describing an organized hierarchy of dimensions of psychological problems that will help us understand their nature by reducing the apparent complexity in them, just like you reduced the complexity of the table full of fruit. We have one more important basis for organizing psychological problems that must be considered, however—the *causes* of psychological problems. The correlations among every dimension of psychological problems are informative because they can help us discover the reasons why every dimension of psychological problems is correlated with every other dimension.[2] When we fully work out what causes these patterns of widespread correlations among every dimension of psychological problems, we will have advanced our understanding of psychological problems to a remarkable degree.

For this reason, my colleagues and I have proposed a formal and testable *causal hypothesis* to stimulate studies that will eventually explain the correlations among every dimension of psychological problems.[2,18,26,32] Specifically, we posited that all dimensions of psychological problems are correlated in a hierarchical manner because there is not only a hierarchy of correlations but also a *hierarchy of causes* of these problems—and a corresponding hierarchy of the psychological and biological mechanisms through which the causal influences operate.[2,4,18] Examination of this hypothesis in some detail is needed because this part of the thesis of this book does represent a radical departure from the thinking underlying the diagnostic categories in the DSM. As all hypotheses in science, our radical proposal is falsifiable. This means that empirical tests can easily tell us if it is partly or entirely wrong. If the hierarchical hypothesis of causes is supported by future data, however, it will force us to think very differently about the nature

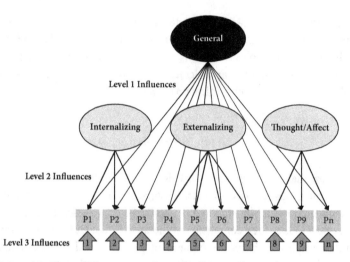

Figure 6.3 Three different sets of causal influences (arrows) are hypothesized to influence every dimension (P1–P*n*) at three different levels of specificity.

of psychological problems. In particular, it will put an end to the un-supportable idea that each "mental disorder" is a discrete entity with its own unique causes.

Specifically, the causal hierarchy proposes that the causes of psycho-logical problems operate in a hierarchy of *shared causes* that has at least three levels.[2]

Level 1: Highly Nonspecific Causal Influences
As illustrated in Figure 6.3, the first level of the proposed causal hi-erarchy consists of causal risk factors that are *highly nonspecific*.[†] This means that some of the things that cause psychological problems are hypothesized to *nonspecifically* increase the risk of having *some* kind of psychological problem, but not *which* kind of problem the person will

---

[†] I'm not doing this just to keep you on your toes! The most nonspecific causal influences on psychological problems that are associated with the general factor are portrayed at the *top* of Figure 6.3 for ease of interpretation. The general factor is at the *bottom* of Figure 6.2, which portrays dimensions of psychological problems, not levels of the causes of those problems as portrayed in Figure 6.3.

experience.[2,33] This hypothesis alone is a radical departure from how we have previously thought about each mental disorder as having its own causes.

Much remains to be learned about the causes that operate at this level, but it appears that some important "familial" risk factors exert their influences at Level 1 of the causal hierarchy. By this I mean that there is now strong evidence that robust genetic risk factors that are passed from one generation of the family to the next, and some aspects of the environment that are common to the entire family, such as poverty and adversity, operate in nonspecific ways at the first level of causal hiearchy.[2,34–36] This would explain why psychological problems are well known to "run in families" but not to "breed true." This means that although parents who meet diagnostic criteria for each kind of mental disorder are more likely to have children who also meet criteria for some kind of mental disorder, it can be any mental disorder, not just the same problem that the parent has.[37] This is likely to be the case because some familial genetic and environmental causes are entirely nonspecific and not linked to any particular dimension of psychological problems.

Notably, however, familial influences are not entirely nonspecific. An important nuance is that many studies indicate that the nonspecific causal influences operating at Level 1 of the causal hierarchy influence risk for each dimension of psychological problems to different degrees. For example, the likelihood of exhibiting specific phobias—intense fears of specific objects or situations, such as snakes or heights—seems to be only modestly increased by the highly nonspecific genetic and environmental influences that operate at Level 1, whereas the likelihood of problems of depression and generalized anxiety is more strongly related to these highly nonspecific causal factors.[2] Thus, the nonspecific causal factors that operate at Level 1 to increase the risk for every form of psychological problems increase the risk of some problems more than others.

The first and many subsequent studies that supported the hypothesis of highly nonspecific genetic and familial environmental factors that influence every dimension of psychological problems through Level 1 of the causal hierarchy were investigations of twins.[2,18,35,38] As discussed in more detail in Chapter 8, twin studies allow inferences regarding the genetic and environmental influences on psychological problems owing to the differences in the genetic relatedness of the two kinds of twins: identical twins, which arise from a single fertilized egg and have essentially identical DNA sequences, and fraternal twins, which develop from two separate fertilized eggs and are no more similar in their DNA sequences than ordinary siblings born at different times—50% similarity on average. If certain assumptions are met, twin studies allow us to estimate the extent to which multiple dimensions of psychological problems are influenced by the same genetic variants, without actually measuring those DNA variants.[39] The logic is straightforward: If the correlation between, for example, conduct problems and ADHD is greater across the members of identical twin pairs than across members of fraternal twin pairs, we can infer that the higher correlation is a result of the much greater similarity in DNA sequences in identical than fraternal twins.[18,39] We can draw this inference with a good degree of confidence because both kinds of twins were born at the same time into the same families and communities. Such studies have revealed that each dimension is correlated with every other dimension more strongly in identical than fraternal twins, suggesting a highly nonspecific contribution of some genetic factors to the risk for any dimension of psychological problems.[18] A massive study of 3 million full- and half-siblings, which also differ in their degrees of genetic similarity, reached the same conclusion.[38]

More recent studies have used molecular genetic methods to examine the same hypothesis. In these studies, variations in DNA are directly measured in cells obtained from blood or saliva from each person so that associations between variants in DNA sequences and different kinds of psychological problems can be identified.[40] Evidence from recent large molecular genetic studies has revealed that many variants in the DNA sequence are nonspecifically associated with the risk for many different forms of psychological problems.[33,40–42] This is very encouraging because all three scientific strategies that provide evidence on causes of psychological problems (i.e., twins, siblings, and DNA studies) consistently indicate widespread sharing of highly nonspecific—also known as pleiotropic—genetic risk factors across different kinds of psychological problems.[2,33,43] Again, this evidence is entirely inconsistent with the DSM diagnostic approach that each "mental disorder" is a qualitatively distinct entity with its own unique causes. Psychological problems cannot be qualitatively distinct in their biological and psychological natures if they share some of the same causal influences.[44]

Even stronger molecular studies of psychological problems are needed for several reasons, however. Only a few kinds of psychological problems have been studied to date, and these molecular genetic studies have consistently used DSM diagnoses rather than dimensional measures. In addition, currently published studies mostly have used "case–control" methods in which persons who meet criteria for a particular mental disorder are recruited in clinics and then compared to persons without that mental disorder who were recruited in very different ways. Such case–control studies likely distort the correlations among psychological problems relative to studies of samples that represent the entire population of people. Nonetheless, the fact that these different scientific strategies for studying genetic influences, which are based on very different methods and assumptions, reach roughly the same conclusions about highly nonspecific genetic risk factors is very encouraging that we are on the right track.

Although current evidence suggests that most of the broadly shared Level 1 causal influences on psychological problems that make them correlated are genetic or environmental factors that are common to all family members, there is evidence that some specific experiences that occur to only one member of a family also might increase risk for any kind of psychological problems in nonspecific ways. In particular, there is evidence the experience of being maltreated in childhood nonspecifically increases risk for every kind of psychological problem.[12,45]

Level 2: Partially Nonspecific Causal Influences

In addition to the broadly nonspecific genetic and environmental causes of psychological problems that operate at Level 1 of the hierarchy of causes, there is robust evidence that at least one additional level of nonspecific causal factors is part of the causal hierarchy. At Level 2 of the hypothesized causal hierarchy shown in Figure 6.3, a number of separate sets of genetic and environmental risk are hypothesized to nonspecifically increase risk for any and all dimensions within each of several subsets of highly correlated psychological problems—meaning the second-order dimensions. These nonspecific causal risk factors are separate from the ones that operate at Level 1 and are distinguished from them by influencing only the dimensions of psychological problems in a single second-order domain, like all internalizing or all externalizing dimension, but not other dimensions. The number of such subsets of dimensions of psychological problems that need to be distinguished is currently unknown, but Level 2 of the causal hierarchy is illustrated in Figure 6.3 based on educated guesses that are based on current evidence.[2,12,27]

Thus, it is reasonable to hypothesize that some of the causal factors that operate at Level 2 nonspecifically influence the likelihood of any and all of the *internalizing* dimensions of psychological problems defined previously, but only the internalizing dimensions. Similarly, it is almost certain that another separate set of genetic and environmental risk factors nonspecifically increases risk for any and all of the *externalizing* dimensions of psychological problems to varying extents.[34] A review of the results of many twin and sibling studies supported the view that the various dimensions within only the internalizing domain and within only the externalizing domain are separate from one another and separate from Level 1 causal factors.[2] That is, it is good evidence that dimensions within the internalizing and externalizing domains share genetic influences over and above the genetic influences that are shared among all dimensions of psychological problems at Level 1 in the causal hierarchy.[34] The same is hypothesized to be true for the dimensions in the second-order domain of psychotic problems of thought and affect, but fewer studies have been conducted to evaluate that part of the hypothesis.[41,46] Nonetheless, it appears likely that one set of genetic and environmental factors is shared at Level 1 and two or more different sets of genetic and environmental factors are shared at Level 2.

Level 3: Dimension-Specific Causal Influences

At the third level of the hypothesized causal hierarchy, there are causal factors that increase risk of only a single dimension of psychological problem (e.g., depression or compulsive rituals). Whereas the genetic and environmental risk factors that operate at Levels 1 and 2 of the causal hierarchy cause dimensions to be correlated, the dimension-specific genetic and environmental risk factors that operate at Level 3 are *unique* to each dimension and *differentiate* one dimension from another. Unlike the causal influences at Levels 1 and 2, they influence an individual's risk only for that particular dimension of psychological problems and do not contribute to the correlations that we see among dimensions. These will almost certainly include some genetic influences that are specific to each dimension and some experiences that are unique to each person in a family.[2,34] A remarkable recent paper reported, however, that the percent of statisitically significant genetic variants that were associated with only one mental disorder ranged from 0% to 27% for each of a half dozen disorders. For example, only 5 of the 40 genetic variants that were found to be associated with depression were specific to only depression. The other 35 variants also were associated with other disorders.[47] Thus, there is converging evidence from both twin and molecular genetic studies that most of the genetic influences on psychological problems are non-specific. We need more evidence, however, and whether these genetic influences are shared at Level 1 or 2 of the causal hierarchy.

It is entirely possible that more than the three levels of causal influences shown in Figure 6.3 will be discovered. Time and huge amounts of new data will tell, but the thrust of the model would remain the same no matter how many levels are eventually discovered: The notion that each "mental disorder" distinguished in the DSM has only its own distinct causes can be ruled out; the causes of dimensions of psychological problems are both substantially shared with one another (at Levels 1 and 2) and unique (at Level 3). That is one of the key take-home messages of this book.

Direct and Indirect Sharing of Causal Influences

The hypotheses stated in this chapter about how causal influences are shared by dimensions of psychological problems represent the best guesses of a number of scientists.[2,27] There is a sensible alternative explanation for the sharing of nonspecific genetic and environmental influences that must not be excluded from further study, however. Let us consider a genetic variant that influences multiple dimensions of psychological problems. Instead of that genetic variant directly influencing all of these dimensions of psychological problems—we will call them dimensions x, y, and z—it is possible that the genetic variant increases risk for x, which then indirectly increases risk for y and z.[48-50] It seems likely to me that some of this kind of indirect sharing of causal influences does occur. For example, there is evidence that persons with high levels of externalizing problems, such as ADHD and antisocial behavior, suffer adverse consequences as a result of their behavior—for example, the alienation of peers, school expulsion, job loss, and incarceration—and that these adverse consequences then increase their likelihood of depression.[51,52] In this case, the causal influences on externalizing problems are shared with depression indirectly through the adverse consequences of the externalizing behavior. Thus, the sharing of causal influences may very well operate through both direct and indirect pathways. It will be important to work out such causal pathways, as this may give us a way to, for example, reduce depression by reducing externalizing problems. The important point, however, is that a large proportion of causal influences are shared by multiple dimensions of psychological problems one way or another. This is fundamental to an improved understanding of psychological problems: They are all correlated because they share causes. Find the shared causes and we can substantially reduce the prevalence of many or all dimensions of psychological problems.

Why Are There Many Different Kinds of Psychological Problems?

The causal hierarchy hypothesis just described provides an explanation for why the many dimensions of psychological problems are robustly correlated. Because nonspecific risk factors operating at Levels 1 and 2 influence multiple forms of psychopathology in the same direction— directly or indirectly—they necessarily result in correlations among the various kinds of psychological problems. Okay, but if causal influences are strongly shared, why is there not just one dimension of psychological problem? In other words, it may help for us to stand the causal model advocated in this book on its head and ask, What *differentiates* dimensions of psychological problems?

I have already provided some answers, but let us address the issue again by focusing on the three levels of the causal hierarchy. Although it appears that the majority of genetic influences are broadly shared by multiple dimensions of psychological problems at the first and second levels of the hierarchy in Figure 6.3, there also are some genetic influences that are unique to each specific dimension of psychological problems at the third level.[2,34] The same is true for the family environment, meaning those experiences that are shared by all members of the same family, such as living in poverty or in a dysfunctional and violent neighborhood. The influence of the family environment is mostly shared by multiple dimensions of psychological problems at Level 1 and Level 2. Still, dimension-specific familial factors operating at the second and third levels of the hierarchy are one reason why there is not just one dimension of psychological problems.

Nonetheless, it appears that the primary driver of *differentiation*—the main reason that there is more than one dimension of psychological problem—is the environmental events that are unique to each individual in a family. I am referring to experiences such as only one sibling going to college, joining the military, or being the victim of a violent crime. What we get from our family is mostly nonspecific influences on our likelihood of exhibiting *some kind* of psychological problem, but what happens to us as individuals plays an important role in which *specific kind* of problems we experience. Looked at from a broader perspective, environmental influences at the individual level play an important role in differentiating the broad variety of different, albeit correlated, dimensions of psychological problems describe in Chapters 3–5.

By the same token, it is our individual experiences that probably influence most of the *changes* that we experience in our psychological problems over time. As we move through our lives, at times gracefully but often stumblingly, many of the causes of our psychological problems do not change. Our family history does not change—all our lives, we will remain children who grew up in a particular neighborhood. Similarly, the sequences of nucleotides in our DNA do not change. Those factors will continue to influence our likelihood of experiencing psychological problems all our lives. Nonetheless, the *expression* of our genes can change, and that is influenced by the changing experiences that are unique to us as individuals. In that and other ways, our own unfolding experiences impact how our psychological problems wax and wane over time. This may result in change from one dimension of problems to another, the disappearance of all problems, or the emergence of new problems.

There are likely to be limits on how much each of us will change over time, however. Our changing experiences can change us, but because the enduring nonspecific causal influences at Levels 1 and 2 in Figure 6.3 are robust, changes in our psychological problems are constrained by our genetic and environmental influences. In other words, the unchanging genetic and familial factors that operate at all levels of the causal hierarchy appear to explain why the changes in our psychological problems typically do not stray far. That is, a person is more likely to change from one psychological problem to another with which it shares more enduring genetic and familial influences.[53] For example, there is evidence that specific phobias and social anxiety share many of their causal influences.[18] Specific phobias and conduct problems—manipulative lying, theft, aggression, and vandalism—share their causal influences to a lesser extent.[18] Thus, it makes sense that persons exhibiting a specific phobia during one year of life may have an increased likelihood of experiencing marked social anxiety 2 years later, and vice versa. In contrast, persons who exhibit a specific phobia are only slightly more likely than chance to begin to engage in antisocial behavior 2 years later; they do not share enough of their nonspecific causal influences for this transition to be common. Thus, according to the current hypothesis, our experiences change and differentiate our psychological problems, but they do so within the constraints created by the causal influences that are shared by multiple dimensions of psychological problems at multiple levels.[2,53]

References

1. Kotov R, Krueger RF, Watson D. A paradigm shift in psychiatric classification: The Hierarchical Taxonomy of Psychopathology (HiTOP). *World Psychiatry*. 2018;17(1):24–25.

2. Lahey BB, Krueger RF, Rathouz PJ, Waldman ID, Zald DH. A hierarchical causal taxonomy of psychopathology across the life span. *Psychological Bulletin.* 2017;143:142–186.

3. Achenbach TM, Conners CK, Quay HC, Verhulst FC, Howell CT. Replication of empirically derived syndromes as a basis for taxonomy of child and adolescent psychopathology. *Journal of Abnormal Child Psychology.* 1989;17:299–323.

4. Lahey BB, Applegate B, Hakes JK, Zald DH, Hariri AR, Rathouz PJ. Is there a general factor of prevalent psychopathology during adulthood? *Journal of Abnormal Psychology.* 2012;121(4):971–977.

5. Lahey BB, Applegate B, Waldman ID, Loft JD, Hankin BL, Rick J. The structure of child and adolescent psychopathology: Generating new hypotheses. *Journal of Abnormal Psychology.* 2004;113:358–385.

6. Watson D, O'Hara MW, Stuart S. Hierarchical structures of affect and psychopathology and their implications for the classification of emotional disorders. *Depression and Anxiety.* 2008;25:282–288.

7. Ivanova MY, Achenbach TM, Rescorla LA, et al. Syndromes of self-reported psychopathology for ages 18–59 in 29 societies. *Journal of Psychopathology and Behavioral Assessment.* 2015;37(2):171–183.

8. Krueger RF, Markon KE, Patrick CJ, Iacono WG. Externalizing psychopathology in adulthood: A dimensional–spectrum conceptualization and its implications for DSM-V. *Journal of Abnormal Psychology.* 2005;114:537–550.

9. Lahey BB, Zald DH, Perkins SF, et al. Measuring the hierarchical general factor model of psychopathology in young adults. *International Journal of Methods in Psychiatric Research.* 2018;27:e1593.

10. Achenbach TM, Becker A, Dopfner M, et al. Multicultural assessment of child and adolescent psychopathology with ASEBA and SDQ instruments: Research findings, applications, and future directions. *Journal of Child Psychology and Psychiatry.* 2008;49:251–275.

11. Carragher N, Teesson M, Sunderland NC, et al. The structure of adolescent psychopathology: A symptom-level analysis. *Psychological Medicine.* 2016;46:981–994.

12. Caspi A, Houts RM, Belsky DW, et al. The p factor: One general psychopathology factor in the structure of psychiatric disorders? *Clinical Psychological Science.* 2014;2:119–137.

13. Angold A, Costello EJ. Puberty and depression. *Child and Adolescent Psychiatric Clinics of North America.* 2006;15:919–937.

14. Clark LA, Watson D, Reynolds S. Diagnosis and classification of psychopathology: Challenges to the current system and future directions. *Annual Review of Psychology.* 1995;46:121–153.

15. Krueger RF, Markon KE. Reinterpreting comorbidity: A model-based approach to understanding and classifying psychopathology. *Annual Review of Clinical Psychology.* 2006;2:111–133.

16. Spearman C. "General intelligence" objectively determined and measured. *American Journal of Psychology.* 1904;15:201–292.
17. Jones EA. A valedictory address. *International Journal of Psychoanalysis.* 1946;27:7–12.
18. Lahey BB, Van Hulle CA, Singh AL, Waldman ID, Rathouz PJ. Higher-order genetic and environmental structure of prevalent forms of child and adolescent psychopathology. *Archives of General Psychiatry.* 2011;68:181–189.
19. Lahey BB, Rathouz PJ, Keenan K, Stepp SD, Loeber R, Hipwell AE. Criterion validity of the general factor of psychopathology in a prospective study of girls. *Journal of Child Psychology and Psychiatry.* 2015;4:415–422.
20. Laceulle OM, Chung JM, Vollebergh WAM, Ormel J. The wide-ranging life outcome correlates of a general psychopathology factor in adolescent psychopathology. *Personality and Mental Health.* 2020;14(1):9–29.
21. Pettersson E, Lahey BB, Lundström S, Larsson H, Lichtenstein P. Criterion validity and utility of the general factor of psychopathology in childhood: Predictive associations with independently measured severe adverse mental health outcomes in adolescence. *Journal of the American Academy of Child and Adolescent Psychiatry.* 2018;57:372–383.
22. O'Reilly LM, Pettersson E, Quinn PD, et al. The association between general childhood psychopathology and adolescent suicide attempt and self-harm: A prospective, population-based twin study. *Journal of Abnormal Psychology.* 2020;129(4):364–375.
23. Conway CC, Forbes MK, Forbush KT, et al. A hierarchical taxonomy of psychopathology can transform mental health research. *Perspectives on Psychological Science.* 2019;14(3):419–436.
24. Forbes MK, Kotov R, Ruggero CJ, Watson D, Zimmerman M, Krueger RF. Delineating the joint hierarchical structure of clinical and personality disorders in an outpatient psychiatric sample. *Comprehensive Psychiatry.* 2017;79:19–30.
25. Krueger RF, Kotov R, Watson D, et al. Progress in achieving quantitative classification of psychopathology. *World Psychiatry.* 2018;17(3):282–293.
26. Lahey BB, Krueger RF, Rathouz PJ, Waldman ID, Zald DH. Perspective: Validity and utility of the general factor of psychopathology. *World Psychiatry.* 2017;16:142–143.
27. Caspi A, Moffitt TE. All for one and one for all: Mental disorders in one dimension. *American Journal of Psychiatry.* 2018;175(9):831–844.
28. Kotov R, Krueger RF, Watson D, et al. The Hierarchical Taxonomy of Psychopathology (HiTOP): A dimensional alternative to traditional nosologies. *Journal of Abnormal Psychology.* 2017;126(4):454–477.
29. Moore TM, Kaczkurkin AN, Durham EL, et al. Criterion validity and relationships between alternative hierarchical dimensional models of general and specific psychopathology. *Journal of Abnormal Psychology.* 2020;129(7):677–688.

30. Brandes CM, Herzhoff K, Smack AJ, Tackett JL. The p factor and the n factor: Associations between the general factors of psychopathology and neuroticism in children. *Clinical Psychological Science.* 2019;7(6):1266–1284.

31. Caspi A, Houts RM, Ambler A, et al. Longitudinal assessment of mental health disorders and comorbidities across 4 decades among participants in the Dunedin Birth Cohort Study. *JAMA Network Open.* 2020;3(4).

32. Zald DH, Lahey BB. Implications of the hierarchical structure of psychopathology for psychiatric neuroimaging. *Biological Psychiatry.* 2017;2(4):310–317.

33. Smoller JW, Andreassen OA, Edenberg HJ, Faraone SV, Glatt SJ, Kendler KS. Psychiatric genetics and the structure of psychopathology. *Molecular Psychiatry.* 2019;24:409–420.

34. Waldman ID, Poore HE, van Hulle C, Rathouz PJ, Lahey BB. External validity of a hierarchical dimensional model of child and adolescent psychopathology: Tests using confirmatory factor analyses and multivariate behavior genetic analyses. *Journal of Abnormal Psychology.* 2016;125(8):1053–1066.

35. Allegrini AG, Cheesman R, Rimfeld K, et al. The p factor: Genetic analyses support a general dimension of psychopathology in childhood and adolescence. *Journal of Child Psychology and Psychiatry.* 2020;61(1):30–39.

36. Selzam S, Coleman JRI, Caspi A, Moffitt TE, Plomin R. A polygenic p factor for major psychiatric disorders. *Translational Psychiatry.* 2018;8(1):205.

37. McLaughlin KA, Gadermann AM, Hwang I, et al. Parent psychopathology and offspring mental disorders: results from the WHO World Mental Health Surveys. *British Journal of Psychiatry.* 2012;200(4):290–299.

38. Pettersson E, Larsson H, Lichtenstein P. Common psychiatric disorders share the same genetic origin: A multivariate sibling study of the Swedish population. *Molecular Psychiatry.* 2016;21:717–721.

39. Neale MC, Cardon LR. *Methodology for genetic studies of twins and families.* Boston: Kluwer; 1992.

40. Selzam S, Coleman JRI, Caspi A, Moffitt TE, Plomin R. A polygenic p factor for major psychiatric disorders. *Translational Psychiatry.* 2018;8(1):205.

41. Smoller JW, Craddock N, Kendler K, et al. Identification of risk loci with shared effects on five major psychiatric disorders: A genome-wide analysis. *Lancet.* 2013;381:1371–1379.

42. Smoller JW, Andreassen OA, Edenberg HJ, Faraone SV, Glatt SJ, Kendler KS. Psychiatric genetics and the structure of psychopathology. *Molecular Psychiatry.* 2019;24(3):409–420.

43. Grotzinger AD, Rhemtulla M, de Vlaming R, et al. Genomic structural equation modelling provides insights into the multivariate genetic architecture of complex traits. *Nature Human Behaviour.* 2019;3(5):513–525.

44. Kendler KS. A gene for . . .: The nature of gene action in psychiatric disorders. *American Journal of Psychiatry.* 2005;162:1243–1252.

45. Weissman DG, Bitran D, Miller AB, Schaefer JD, Sheridan MA, McLaughlin KA. Difficulties with emotion regulation as a transdiagnostic mechanism linking child maltreatment with the emergence of psychopathology. *Development and Psychopathology.* 2019;31(3):899–915.

46. Lichtenstein P, Yip BH, Bjork C, et al. Common genetic determinants of schizophrenia and bipolar disorder in Swedish families: A population-based study. *Lancet.* 2009;373(9659):234–239.

47. Byrne EM, Zhu Z, Qi T, Skene NG, Bryois J, Pardinas AF, . . . Major Depressive Disorder Working Group of the Psychiatric Genomics Consortium (in press). Conditional GWAS analysis to identify disorder-specific SNPs for psychiatric disorders. *Molecular Psychiatry.* doi:10.1038/s41380-020-0705-9

48. Borsboom D, Cramer AOJ. Network analysis: An integrative approach to the structure of psychopathology. *Annual Review of Clinical Psychology.* 2013;9:91–121.

49. Zachar P, Kendler KS. The philosophy of nosology. *Annual Review of Clinical Psychology.* 2017;13:49–71.

50. Abecasis GR, Cardon LR, Cookson WOC. A general test of association for quantitative traits in nuclear families. *American Journal of Human Genetics.* 2000;66:279–292.

51. Patterson GR, Capaldi DM. A mediational model for boys' depressed mood. In: Rolf JE, ed. *Risk and protective factors in the development of psychopathology.* New York: Cambridge University Press; 1990:141–163.

52. Beauchaine TP, Ben-David I, Bos M. ADHD, financial distress, and suicide in adulthood: A population study. *Science Advances.* 2020;6(40).

53. Lahey BB, Zald DH, Hakes JK, Krueger RF, Rathouz PJ. Patterns of heterotypic continuity associated with the cross-sectional correlational structure of prevalent mental disorders in adults. *JAMA Psychiatry.* 2014;71:989–996.

7

Sex Differences and the Dynamic Development of Psychological Problems

This chapter briefly tells the story of the dynamic changes over time in psychological problems among girls and boys, women and men, as we march, bumble, stumble—and sometimes happily sail—through life. It is a story that is fundamentally important but cannot yet be based entirely on sound scientific evidence. Because of the limited current state of our knowledge, I sometimes need to rely on incomplete evidence. Most current evidence comes from relatively weak but quick and inexpensive *cross-sectional studies*, in which different people of different ages are studied at one point in time. Such studies are useful, but they only give us a momentary "snapshot" view of human lives at different ages. These snapshots can tell us something about psychological problems at different ages, but they cannot tell us how each person's problems change over time. As a result, it is difficult to see that psychological problems are constantly changing aspects of lives that unfold over long periods of time. Moreover, we have to be careful in our interpretation of cross-sectional studies because they are based on different people at different ages. If the participants in the study at each age are not exactly comparable, any apparent age difference might be inaccurate. If professors at age 30 years were tested on arm strength and compared to professional body builders at age 40 years, we might erroneously conclude that arm strength increases over that decade.

Cross-sectional studies are valuable, however, in generating hypotheses about developmental change that can be tested in stronger but more expensive and lengthy *longitudinal studies.* Longitudinal studies examine the same persons repeatedly over time, often for many years, allowing us to see changes in these individuals as they develop. Unfortunately, fewer longitudinal studies of adequately large and representative samples have been conducted.

Crucially, it is impossible to consider developmental change in psychological problems without simultaneously considering the equally important topic of sex differences.* Conversely, we cannot think about sex differences without considering developmental differences—these two topics are inextricably intertwined. This is because the age differences in many dimensions of psychological problem are different in females and males, and differences between the sexes in psychological problems are not the same at different ages.

Although the current evidence on sex and age differences in psychological problems is not nearly as complete as we need it to be, a reasonably accurate—if tentative—picture can be pieced together from the cross-sectional and longitudinal studies that have been published to date. One challenge in doing so is that the information we most need can only come from the limited number of studies that examined both age and sex differences together. Another important limitation is that almost every published study on sex and age differences has used *Diagnostic and Statistical Manual of Mental Disorders* (DSM) categorical diagnoses rather than continuous measures of dimensions of psychological problems. Thus, I can paint a fuzzy but hopefully still useful picture of sex differences and developmental change using the available data. Keep in mind that this chapter may include inaccurate statements that will be revealed by better studies in the future.

Every kind of psychological problem occurs in both females and males, and the sexes are about equally likely to experience some kind

---

* I use the term sex in this chapter because nearly all published studies asked people to classify themselves in a binary way on the basis of their "sex." We have little evidence in the field of psychological problems on persons whose biological sex is ambiguous or persons who identify with a different gender, multiple genders, or no gender at all. It is entirely possible that the generalizations about sex differences described in this chapter do not apply to everyone. Not enough is yet known about these important issues.

of psychological problem. They are not equally likely to experience the *same kinds* of psychological problems, however. Most dimensions of psychological problems are more common in one sex than in the other. Similarly, although most psychological problems can be found in persons of any age, each dimension of psychological problems is considerably more common at some ages than others.

Why are these sex and age differences important? For one thing, understanding sex and age differences in psychological problems is fundamental to understanding the experiences of female and male children, adolescents, and adults across their lives. If we carefully keep in mind that we are only talking about average differences among the sexes and age groups that do not apply to every individual, and we are scrupulously careful to avoid stereotyping by never assuming that every individual is like the average for their group, then the information in this chapter can help us understand and appreciate the diversity of human lives.

In addition, sex and age differences are important simply because they are often quite large. When we discover the powerful causes of age and sex differences, we will have learned a great deal about the causes of psychological problems per se. For example, there is a steady and ultimately large increase in the number of persons who experience depression that begins during late adolescence and extends into early middle age. What biological changes and/or changes in experiences around this time cause this increase in depression? Why does it start during late adolescence instead of some other time in life? Furthermore, what causes this increase in depression to be steeper in females? And why do women continue to experience depression for the first time in their lives over more years than men? We cannot achieve a full understanding of the causes of psychological problems until we have answers to these and similar questions about all forms of psychological problems.

Psychological Problems across Our Lives

In this section, I summarize what is known about developmental changes in psychological problems from early childhood through later adulthood, distinguishing between developmental changes in females and males. I describe changes separately in the three broad domains of psychological problems described in Chapters 3–5:internalizing, externalizing, and psychotic problems. Keep in mind, however, that all dimensions of psychological problems are correlated, both within and among these three domains, which means that we rarely experience just one kind of psychological problem at a time. That is not to say, however, that all dimensions of psychological problems exhibit the same sex and age differences; they most definitely do not.

Incidence, Prevalence, and Age of Onset

I have been using the term *prevalence* to refer to the proportion of persons in a population who have a problem during some period of time, such as during the past 12 months. To fully understand how psychological problems change with increasing age, however, we also need the concept of *incidence.* This is the proportion of persons in a population who exhibit a given problem for the *first time* in their life at a particular age. The related term of *age of onset* is the average age of the incidence of each kind of problem.

There has long been evidence that an earlier age of onset of conduct problems (i.e., during childhood instead of during adolescence) is associated with greater severity and perhaps a greater likelihood of persistence of antisocial behavior into adulthood.[1] In contrast, youth who were well-behaved children and engage in antisocial behavior for the first time after puberty usually engage in only relatively minor problem behaviors, such as truancy, shoplifting, and lying to parents, and they usually desist from their youthful antisocial behavior as they make the transition to adulthood.[2] There is increasingly strong evidence that an earlier age of onset could be important to many different dimensions of psychological problems in the same way. Recent evidence suggests that persons who develop most kinds of psychological problems earlier in life generally have more serious and more long-lasting psychological problems of all sorts compared with persons who develop new problems in late adolescence or early adulthood.[3-5]

Changes in Psychological Problems during Childhood

Although we usually think of psychological problems as being something that adults experience, some children begin their lives as troubled toddlers. Indeed, several dimensions of psychological problems begin at very early ages. Although very few toddlers meet DSM criteria for conduct disorder, for example, they are not quite the innocents we usually consider them to be. Hitting, kicking, biting, and taking things from others are pretty common by 18–24 months of age, with little difference between girls and boys in the prevalence of these behaviors during toddlerhood.[6] All told, something on the order of 20% of preschool children meet DSM criteria for at least one mental disorder, and many more have psychological problems that do not quite reach those thresholds.[7-9] These early childhood psychological problems are not insignificant phenomena; young children with psychological problems are at increased risk for serious future psychological problems and impaired functioning in adolescence and adulthood.[10-14] This important topic is discussed more in-depth later in this chapter.

Childhood Externalizing Problems

The several specific dimensions of externalizing problems differ considerably in their developmental trends. Oppositional defiant behavior and aggressive conduct problems change very little in prevalence across childhood and early adolescence. In contrast, problems of hyperactivity and impulsivity tend to decline in both sexes with increasing age across childhood and adolescence.[15] Problems in maintaining attention tend to increase in early elementary school, probably because the children's capacity for sustaining attention is first challenged by schoolwork at that time, but this initial increase is followed by very slow declines across childhood and adolescence.[14,16]

In contrast, the prevalence of serious conduct problems increases gradually across childhood and then increases rapidly during adolescence, particularly in youth who display attention-deficit/hyperactivity disorder (ADHD) and oppositional defiant behavior.[17-19] In particular, property crimes (e.g., theft) and status offenses (e.g., truancy) increase from childhood into adolescence.[20] From age 4 or 5 years onward, such conduct problems are more common on average in boys than girls.[6,21-24] These increasingly common problems are quite significant, and young adults who had high levels of conduct problems during childhood are at substantial risk for poor functioning, antisocial behavior, and unhappy lives.[25]

Childhood Internalizing Problems

Problems involving fear often begin in toddlerhood and the preschool period. Specific fears and separation anxiety are the most common internalizing problems in early childhood, but social fears, agoraphobic fears, and generalized worry also are found in young children.[8,26,27] From the preschool years into adolescence, girls are more likely than boys to experience distressing and impairing fears and separation anxiety.[27-33] Childhood fears and separation anxiety decline steeply with increasing age from childhood to adolescence in both sexes, but they do not always go away entirely.[10,14,16,30,34-37]

Fears are more common in females across the life span. In contrast, generalized anxiety and depression are initially slightly more common in boys than girls during childhood, but females show steeper increases during adolescence and early adulthood. Recall from Chapter 3 that worry and depression are highly correlated and are sometimes referred to as "worry–misery" dimensions to distinguish them from fears. The facts that the fears and worry–misery dimensions exhibit both distinct sex differences and age-related changes across childhood are important ways in which these subsets of internalizing dimensions differ.

It is important to mention that fears and worry are not always easy to identify in children. At early ages, internalizing problems often come to the attention of parents and pediatricians when children complain of stomachaches, headaches, and joint pains, which are correlated with internalizing problems.[10]

Autism Spectrum Problems

Autism spectrum problems begin in very early childhood and nearly always endure throughout life. A substantial number of children with autism spectrum problems show improved functioning with increasing age, but they continue to exhibit impairing problems throughout their lives in nearly all cases.[38] In recent years, the scope of what is considered to be autism spectrum problems has been expanded considerably to include milder problems in persons with average or better intelligence. In such individuals, their problems in social interaction may not become evident until school age, when social interactions with persons outside the family become more common. We know little about the life course of such children with milder autism spectrum problems because they have not been studied extensively until recently.

Changes in Psychological Problems during the Transition to Adulthood

During a span of about a decade, from adolescence through early adulthood—approximately 15 through 25 years of age—we make the dramatic transition from children to adolescents to young adults. Caterpillars become butterflies; children become full-grown adults. Keep in mind as you read this section that puberty typically begins earlier in females than males, so the ages at which the transition to adulthood takes place differ by sex. In addition, there is no specific age at which adulthood begins; different people take on the independence and responsibilities of adulthood at different ages. Although the boundaries of the period of transition to adulthood are fuzzy, the dramatic changes in psychological problems that take place then are very clear.

There is some good news about psychological problems during the transition to adulthood that should not be overlooked. Problems of hyperactivity and impulsivity, inattention, and specific fears all continue to decline in prevalence through adolescence and early adulthood.[14,16,20,36] Most of the changes in psychological problems, unfortunately, are in the opposite direction. Sadly, the relatively well-adjusted years at the close of childhood are followed by the start of a steep increase in many serious problems, such as depression, panic attacks, substance use problems, and psychotic problems.[36] Most of the increase in the *prevalence* of psychological problems during adolescence and early adulthood is due to the eruption of new (incident) problems during adolescence and early adulthood. Indeed, adolescence and early adulthood are the peak period of incidence for many kinds of serious psychological problems.[39] These new or worsening psychological problems make the transition to adulthood an extremely difficult time for many youth and also for their families and friends.

Sometimes new psychological problems emerge quite unexpectedly during the transition to adulthood in individuals who had few problems as children. These problems usually do not appear out of the blue, however. The incidence of new psychological problems during the transition to adulthood is more common in persons who had previously experienced other psychological problems as children. That is, many youth change from one dimension of problems to other problems, which is referred to as *heterotypic continuity*. This means that there is continuity in the sense of still having psychological problems over time, but the problems that are experienced change. As I discuss changes in psychological problems during the transition to adulthood, I will mention many common heterotypic transitions from one dimension of psychological problems in childhood to another dimension in adolescence and adulthood. This is a big part of what I mean when I say that this chapter is about the *development* of psychological problems— they change dynamically over time.

Let me be clear that there is still a lot that we need to learn about heterotypic continuity. Consider the well-establish finding that children who exhibit high levels of conduct problems are at increased risk for developing new substance use problems in late adolescence and early adulthood.[40] I think that means that some enduring psychological characteristics of individuals, such as temperament, are manifested as conduct problems when they living in their home and school environments during childhood, but the same enduring characteristics give rise to substance abuse and dependence when they are living adult lives. That might be an incomplete or even an incorrect explanation, however. It could well be that people who live in chaotic and poorly resourced environments as children tend to live in adverse environments during adulthood. The continuity in their psychological problems may come from the continuity in their adverse environments rather than continuity in their psychological characteristics. Much remains to be learned before we can be sure of an explanation, and of course, more than one explanation may be correct.

Thus, the new psychological problems that are experienced during the transition to adulthood sometimes emerge in persons with no previous history of childhood problems, but more often they are experienced by persons who had previously experienced other childhood psychological problems.[40,41] Not all children who exhibit high levels of psychological problems continue to have problems as adults, however. About one-fourth of children with psychological problems appear to be free of problems and impaired functioning in adulthood.[42] Nonetheless, a solid majority go on to experience some kind of psychological problem that is typical of adolescence and adulthood.[42]

Internalizing Problems

The downward trend in childhood fears is offset by increases during adolescence in generalized anxiety, social anxiety, obsessive–compulsive rituals, agoraphobia, panic attacks, social phobia, disordered eating, and depression.[34,36] The increase in each of these problems is steeper and reaches higher levels in females.[31,34,36,43–50] For example, the incidence of the diagnosis of major depression shows a marked increase beginning in early adolescence, and new depression problems emerge for the first time more frequently in females.[51]

Persons who experience panic attacks and agoraphobic fears for the first time during adolescence and early adulthood are usually persons who had exhibited specific fears and separation anxiety during childhood.[52,53] The childhood problems that tend to precede depression during the transition to adulthood are much broader, however. Incident depression is more likely in persons with a history of childhood problems of anxiety, depression, oppositional defiant behavior, or conduct problems.[54–56]

Externalizing Problems

In both sexes, but particularly in males, there is an increase in the prevalence of mature forms of conduct problems during adolescence—theft, vandalism, breaking and entering, running away from home, and assault—until it reaches a peak in late adolescence. These increases in antisocial behavior often occur in adolescents with a history of childhood externalizing problems, but a substantial number of adolescents who had been well-behaved children engage in (mostly) minor antisocial and (mostly) transient antisocial behavior for the first time during adolescence. If the readers of this book briefly engaged in antisocial behavior during adolescence, it is likely that they followed this relatively benign adolescent-onset pattern.

On average, serious antisocial behavior begins a sharp decline in early adulthood.[20,22,57] Most adolescents who engage in conduct problems during adolescence desist from their antisocial ways in early adulthood, but more than one-third of children with conduct problems that persisted from childhood through adolescence continue to exhibit serious and persistent adult antisocial behavior and often engage in crime at high rates.[1,54] More than half of the serious and violent crimes during adulthood are committed by fewer than 5% of the population, most of whom engaged in conduct problems beginning in childhood and persisted into adulthood.[58,59]

The pattern of behaving in callous and impulsive ways, taking advantage of others, and engaging in criminal behavior during adulthood referred to as antisocial personality disorder in the DSM is more common in males.[60] It is generally considered to be the adult manifestation of childhood conduct problems. Because fewer than half of children with serious conduct problems will meet DSM diagnostic criteria for antisocial personality disorder, however, engaging in conduct problems during childhood certainly does not always predict a lifetime of antisocial behavior.[1,61]

Although they can be quite problematic, much less is known about persons who engage in the other dimensions of externalizing problems described in Chapter 4. Male adults are also more likely to exhibit the serious kinds of callous, self-serving, and manipulative behaviors referred to as narcissistic personality disorder.[51] Not enough solid information is available to know if histrionic personality and borderline personality are more common in one sex than another, however.

During adolescence, a new dimension of externalizing problems emerges for the first time that involves the abuse of, or dependence on, psychoactive substances, meaning any substance that alters mood or perception. This includes nicotine, cannabis, alcohol, cocaine, heroin, and other substances. The use of mind-altering substances is rare in childhood but increases dramatically during late adolescence and early adulthood. Females begin to use and abuse psychoactive substances at earlier ages than males, but there is a steeper increase in substance abuse and dependence in males, reaching higher levels than in females by late adolescence and early adulthood.[62,63] Problems of substance abuse and dependence begin for the first time during adolescence and early adulthood, at least partly because youth first have unsupervised access to alcohol, cannabis, tobacco, and other drugs at these ages. Substance abuse and dependence are considered to be externalizing problems partly because they are more strongly correlated with antisocial behavior during adulthood than with other dimensions of psychological problems, but also because they are more likely to arise in persons who exhibited externalizing problems during childhood.[54,64–66]

Psychotic and Other Problems of Thought and Emotion

The psychotic problems that define schizotypal personality disorder, schizophrenia, and manic behavior almost always arise for the first time during adolescence or early adulthood. Recall from Chapter 5 that this diverse group of uncommon but often serious problems involves cognitive disturbances that put the person "out of touch with reality" and sometimes includes variations in energy levels and in affect—feelings and emotions—that are markedly inconsistent with the situation. The DSM diagnoses associated with this set of dimensions include mania (part of bipolar disorder), schizophrenia, paranoid and schizotypal personality disorders, and autism spectrum disorder. Unfortunately, almost all studies of these problems to date have used only categorical diagnoses.

Problems involving delusions, hallucinations, and/or disorganized emotion or behavior that are serious enough to cause impaired functioning and lead to the diagnosis of schizophrenia are uncommon at all ages, but especially in childhood. The onset of schizophrenia is usually gradual, with the syndrome of problems unfolding over a number of months or years. The likelihood of the first diagnosis of schizophrenia increases sharply in adolescence, reaching a peak at about age 20 years in both sexes, but with somewhat more schizophrenic problems in males that are serious enough to require treatment.[43,44,67] The little available evidence suggests that females in the general population are more likely than males to meet diagnostic criteria for paranoid and schizotypal personality disorders, which also emerge mostly during the transition to adulthood.[51]

There is little solid evidence of sex difference in the prevalence of the diagnosis of bipolar disorder,[48] but females may be slightly more likely to exhibit these problems.[68] Mania usually begins in adolescence or early adulthood, with a peak age of onset around 20 years; fewer persons develop new manic problems after early adulthood.[44,68,69] The age of the first diagnosis of bipolar disorder may be slightly later in females than males.[70]

Psychological Problems during Adulthood

Large studies of adults conducted throughout the world indicate that internalizing problems involving fears and worries are both more common in adult women than men.[48] Specifically, adult women in the general population are more likely than men to experience panic attacks, agoraphobic fears, social anxiety, specific phobias, generalized anxiety, post-traumatic stress disorder (PTSD), social avoidance, and social dependence.[48,51] Indeed, studies using categorical diagnoses indicate that women are about twice as likely to experience generalized anxiety disorder, panic disorder, and specific phobia as men, and they are 50% more likely to meet diagnostic criteria for social anxiety disorder than men.[60]

Similarly, depression is more common during adulthood among women than men.[48,51,71] In terms of the categorical DSM diagnosis of major depressive disorder, adult women are nearly twice as likely as men to meet diagnostic criteria for depression.[72] This does not mean that depression is not a common psychological problem for both sexes—it is—but the causes of this very large sex difference must be discovered to fully understand the causes of depression. The sex difference in depression involves more than just a difference in prevalence. The rise in the number of persons meeting criteria for depression for the first time during adolescence begins later in males, rises more slowly, and does not reach the same high and sustained rate of new cases of depression seen in females across early and middle adulthood.[73-75] Suicide is associated with many kinds of psychological problems but particularly depression. Consistent with the greater prevalence of depression and other internalizing problems in females from adolescence on, females are more likely to think seriously about suicide and to attempt to commit suicide.[76–78] Males, however, are more than three times as likely to kill themselves (https://www.cdc.gov/nchs/products/databriefs/db330.htm). This may be due to the use of more lethal means by males, particularly firearms.[79]

Fortunately, the rise in serious psychological problems during the transition to adulthood soon begins to abate. This improvement is part of a general trend for people to gradually experience fewer intense negative emotions and more positive emotions, on average, as they age through adulthood.[80] The prevalence of almost all DSM diagnoses, from anxiety disorder to antisocial personality disorder, declines somewhat from early adulthood through middle age, then declines even more steeply in later adulthood.[51,81–83] Mania and abuse and dependence on alcohol, cannabis, and other drugs decline rapidly after adolescence, whereas the prevalence of PTSD declines much less rapidly until older age.[51,84] Nicotine dependence is an exception because it shows little decline in prevalence until after age 65 years.[51] Abuse and dependence involving all substances are more common in males across adolescence and adulthood.[60]

Overview of Development

Imagine for a moment that we could construct psychological biographies of 1,000 persons that describe their psychological problems in every year of their lives. Most of the 1,000 biographies would include at least a brief brush with distressing and impairing psychological problems. Recall from previous chapters that the *cumulative proportion* of persons who report problems that met diagnostic criteria for at least one mental disorder during any 12-month period in their lives increases dramatically from about 20% in childhood to about 80% by the time they reach middle adulthood.[85,86] That does not mean that 80% of adults *currently* meet criteria for a mental disorder throughout their lives, but it means that almost everyone will meet DSM criteria for at least one mental disorder at least once in their lives.[3] Some of these 1,000 people would experience just one or two kinds of psychological problems for a relatively short period of time and then cease to have problems. They may have gone through several weeks of depression, found that they were drinking alcohol to the point that it interfered with their lives for 2 years, or were too afraid to fly on airplanes for 6 months. Other individuals would be distressed and impaired by some kind of psychological problem during long stretches of their lives, although not necessarily the same kind of problem every year.[87] As I have been saying, the experience of having psychological problems that are serious enough to be distressing or to interfere with our lives to some extent is quite a common thing. Never having a psychological problem is what is uncommon![3,85]

These biographies would reveal great variety in people's psychological problems over time. Indeed, it is likely that we would see virtually every possible pattern of change in psychological problems as these people lived out their lives.[3,87–89] The patterns of changes would be highly erratic. Psychological problems improve or worsen like the value of the stock market over time, showing long-term trends despite sometimes dramatic short-term ups and downs. For example, a 15-year-long longitudinal study of boys whose parents brought them to child psychology and psychiatry clinics found that the boys' psychological problems waxed and waned over time—they had good years and bad years in terms of the psychological problems they exhibited.[90]

Furthermore, the 1,000 biographies would reveal marked variations among individual in which psychological problems they experienced over time. Some would continue to experience the same problem persistently or intermittently across their lives, some would experience one problem now and shift to another problem later, and many other people would add new problems to their old persisting problems over time.[3,87,89,91,92] There is one bit of good news here: The incidence curves in many studies suggest that nearly all of the fortunate minority of persons who make it to later middle age without experiencing significant psychological problems will never experience them in their later lives.

Causes of Sex and Age Differences in Developing Psychological Problems

What causes some psychological problems to be more common in one sex than the other? Or turning the question around, what protects persons of one sex from developing the kinds of psychological problems that are more common in the other sex? Similarly, what causes the marked age differences in the prevalence of most psychological problems? Why do some childhood problems decline while other become more common with increasing age? Why is there a sudden increase in many serious psychological problems during adolescence and early adulthood? What protects children from developing mania and schizophrenia during childhood, and why is that protection lost in late adolescence? Alternatively, what new risk factors for these problems do children face as they become young adults? These are vitally important questions that are begging to be answered, but at this point we can only tentatively sketch some possible explanations.

Causes of Age Differences

Let us begin with the large age differences in psychological problems. There are three different questions to be answered about the causes of age differences.

First, why do the most common psychological problems that begin in early childhood decline with increasing age? Hyperactivity, inattention, and fears all decline in prevalence as children grow older. What causes these improvements in adaptive psychological functioning with increasing age?[22] Jeff Halperin and Kurt Shulz[93] hypothesized that childhood problems of inattention, hyperactivity, and impulsivity—the problems that define the diagnosis of ADHD—improve as regions in the cerebral cortex involved in the regulation of attention and impulses mature during adolescence. According to this theory, we do not outgrow the underlying causes of ADHD, but we can control our attention, impulsivity, and activity better when the so-called executive control networks of the brain mature. This hypothesis has been supported by a number of studies,[94,95] but it remains just a good hypothesis. I wonder, however, if the maturation of networks involved in the control of attention and emotion in the cerebral cortex might also be part of the explanation for the declines in fears from early childhood into adolescence.

Second, why do conduct problems decrease slightly during childhood, increase rapidly during late adolescence, peak around age 17 or 18 years, and then decline again after late adolescence? The conduct problems that surge in adolescence are mostly misbehaviors such as truancy and staying out after dark without parental permission, but more serious problems also emerge in adolescence, such as running away from home, armed robbery, assault, breaking and entering, murder, and forced sex. Any explanation for these age-related increases in serious conduct problems during adolescence is no more than speculation at this point, but it is possible that these problems increase in prevalence partly because of physical development—bigger and stronger youth are better able to threaten strangers and take their wallets—but I suspect that it is mostly because older children and adolescents spend increasing amounts of time away from close adult supervision. Adolescents may be more likely to engage in more serious antisocial behavior than children partly because they have more freedom to do so. In addition, they have the increased cognitive ability to conceal their antisocial behavior from their parents.

It is possible that serious antisocial behavior declines during adulthood after peaking in late adolescence partly because of maturing executive control mechanisms but perhaps also because many young adults have decreasing amounts of unstructured time when they begin to work for a living or join the military services or enter into domestic relationships. This explanation is debatable, however, as it may only be youth who are already giving up antisocial behavior who are able to work and maintain relationships, whereas more persistently antisocial youth are less successful in jobs or relationships. So desistance from antisocial behavior may be the cause rather that the effect here.

Third, what causes the psychological problems of depression, generalized anxiety, social anxiety, obsessive–compulsive rituals, panic, disordered eating, mania, schizophrenia, and substance use disorders to become (collectively) common for the first time in late adolescence and early adulthood? Because of the marked sex differences in most of these problems, I suggest answers in the next section of this chapter as we discuss the possible causes of sex differences in these problems. Again, we can only speculate about possible answers at this point, keeping in mind that there probably will be more than one answer to each question.

Causes of Sex Differences

Why do the psychological problems that usually begin in childhood typically differ by sex? Why are some problems more common in boys (e.g., ADHD, oppositional defiant behaviors, conduct problems, and autism spectrum problems) and some are more common in girls (e.g., fears)? In addition, why is the spike in conduct problems during adolescence steeper in males but the spike in depression, generalized anxiety, dangerously disordered eating, and other problems is steeper in females? Because brain and behavior are two inseparable sides of the same coin, this almost certainly is related to the rapid changes in the developing brain that occur during this time.[96] The sex differences in the incidence of depression and other problems during the transition to adulthood are likely to be linked to sex differences in the development of the brain during this time of life. What causes these sex differences in brain and behavior? There are two obvious possible causes of sex differences in the development of psychological problems—differences in genetic risks and differences in experiences.

Genetic Factors in Sex Differences

As discussed in detail in Chapter 8, every dimension of psychological problems is influenced by a combination of both environmental and genetic factors. Let us first ask if there are genetic factors that could cause the sex differences in psychological problems? There is only one obvious candidate for the genetic cause of the hypothetical sex difference in thresholds. Sequences of DNA that encode proteins—genes, in other words—are located on the 23 pairs of chromosomes that we inherit from our biological parents. We randomly inherit one chromosome in each of these pairs from each parent. There are no differences between females and males in this random process for 22 of our pairs of chromosomes, so any genetic causes of sex differences are unlikely to be encoded in the DNA of these chromosomes. Nonetheless, there is a clear difference in the 23rd chromosome—the sex chromosome. Females inherit two "X" sex chromosomes and males inherit one "X" and one "Y" sex chromosome.[†] Therefore, differences between the sexes in the sex chromosome could contribute to sex differences in psychological problems.

Crucially, genes on sex chromosomes influence the physical characteristics of the sexes, partly by influencing how other genes are expressed in males and females. This results in sex differences in all parts of the body, including the brain.[97] Our human brains are amazingly fine-tuned instruments in both females and males, but there are sex differences in the development of the brain.[98] These average differences in the brains of females and males certainly do not mean that the brains of one sex are superior to the other, but they are different on average. Because there are sex differences in psychological problems, and every variation in behavior is necessarily accompanied by variations in brain and other bodily systems, this is not surprising.

Thus, one hypothesis is that some of the causes of sex differences in brain and behavior, including psychological problems, are due to the differences between the sexes in the sex chromosome.[99,100] This almost certainly involves not just differences in the proteins encoded by the X and Y chromosomes but also sex differences in the expression of genes that reside on other chromosomes.[101]

Sex Differences in Experience

Sex differences in psychological problems almost definitely also involve differences in gene expression triggered by differences in the experiences of women and men.[98,102] There is no such thing as a typical male or female life, of course, but females and males tend to have different experiences during their lives on average. This begins in the subtly different ways in which parents interact with their female and

---

[†] Again, I am simplifying here because of limitations in the available evidence. There are other combinations of X and Y chromosomes, such as having more than one Y, and sex is not always a binary variable. Furthermore, there are quite often differences between one's sex and the gender with which one identifies.

male infants and continues throughout life. Even today, females in some families are more likely to be encouraged to pursue feminine play, studies, sports, and occupations.[103] Similarly, there are often sex differences in experiences because men are more likely to work in jobs such as construction and mechanics, whereas women are more likely to be employed in service and caring roles.[104]

Particularly relevant to psychological problems are sex differences in stressful experiences. Although males and females both experience stress in their lives, they differ on average in the kinds of stressors they experience. Females are more likely to experience stalking, physical assault by a partner, sexual harassment and discrimination, and sexual predation and assault, whereas males are more likely to be mugged, physically assaulted, suspended from school, and arrested and incarcerated.[105–108] Thus, females and males may exhibit different reactions to stress on average partly because they tend to be exposed to different stressors.

Even when females and males are exposed to exactly the same stressor, however, there are average differences in responses to the stressor by females and males. Consider the horribly stressful experiences of a group of Norwegian youth in 2011.[109] An armed terrorist dressed as a police officer went to a small island off the coast near Oslo, where there was a summer camp for 500 members of a youth organization. He hunted the youth for more than an hour with a gun, killing 69 and injuring more than 100, until a police rescue team arrested him. Understandably, many of the youth experienced depression and post-traumatic stress reactions afterwards. For reasons that are not yet understood, however, female youth were more likely to experience psychological problems after the attack than males. Research to understand sex differences in reactions to stress is a high priority for the field because we will not understand stress reactions until we understand average sex differences in stress reactions.

Sex Protection Hypothesis

This hypothesis provides a somewhat different perspective on sex differences in psychological problems that may be useful. The hypothesis is that something about being female protects most girls from externalizing problems and autism spectrum problems, and conversely, something about being a male protects most boys from fears, worries, and depression.[110] That is, it is possible that the same causes of each dimension of psychological problems have to surpass different thresholds in the two sexes. For example, if a hypothetical protective factor for ADHD exits for females, it would mean that females who display high levels of ADHD problems need higher levels of the genetic and environmental risk factors for ADHD problems than males would need to exhibit the same level of these problems.

A number of studies have supported this sex protection hypothesis, including a large Swedish study of 7,000 pairs of fraternal (i.e., not identical) twins.[111] Some of these fraternal twin pairs were of the same sex and some were of different sexes. Twin pairs were identified in which at least one twin displayed high levels of ADHD problems. One member of these twin pairs was randomly designated to be the "proband" and the other designated the "co-twin." These studies made use of the fact that fraternal twin pairs are of the same age and live in the same family environments during childhood, reducing differences in their experiences. In addition, female and male fraternal twin pairs share their genes to the same extent (except for the sex chromosome). Thus, if there is no protective factor for females in the case of ADHD, the genetic and environmental factors shared by the two members of the twin pairs should result in the co-twin of a proband with serious ADHD problems experiencing the same level of ADHD problems regardless of whether the proband was a female or a male. The result, however, was that the co-twins of female probands with ADHD problems had higher levels of ADHD problems than the co-twins of male probands with ADHD problems. This result supports the hypothesis that female probands must have more of the genes and experiences that cause ADHD to reach a high level of ADHD problems.[111] The sharing of the higher levels of those genetic and environmental risk factors with their co-twin is what caused the higher level of ADHD problems in the co-twins of female probands. Other studies of twins have similarly suggested that something protects females from developing autism spectrum problems and adolescent conduct problems.[112,113] This is one of the many lines of inquiry that remain to be followed to identify the causes of sex and age differences in psychological problems.

References

1. Lahey BB, Loeber R, Burke JD, Applegate B. Predicting future antisocial personality disorder in males from a clinical assessment in childhood. *Journal of Consulting and Clinical Psychology*. 2005;73:389–399.
2. Fairchild G, van Goozen SHM, Calder AJ, Goodyer IM. Research review: Evaluating and reformulating the developmental taxonomic theory of antisocial behaviour. *Journal of Child Psychology and Psychiatry*. 2013;54(9):924–940.
3. Caspi A, Houts RM, Ambler A, et al. Longitudinal assessment of mental health disorders and comorbidities across 4 decades among participants in the Dunedin Birth Cohort Study. *JAMA Network Open*. 2020;3(4):10e203221.
4. De Vries YA, Al-Hamzawi A, Alonso J, et al. Transdiagnostic development of internalizing psychopathology throughout the life course up to age 45: A World Mental Health Surveys report. *Psychological Medicine*. 2020:1–10.
5. Moffitt TE. Psychiatry's opportunity to prevent the rising burden of age-related disease *JAMA Psychiatry*. 2019;76:461–462.
6. Tremblay RE, Japel C, Perusse D, et al. The search for the age of "onset" of physical aggression: Rousseau and Bandura revisited. *Criminal Behaviour and Mental Health*. 1999;9:8–23.
7. Keenan K, Wakschlag LS. More than the terrible twos: The nature and severity of behavior problems in clinic-referred preschool children. *Journal of Abnormal Child Psychology*. 2000;28(1):33–46.
8. Wichstrom L, Berg-Nielsen TS, Angold A, Egger HL, Solheim E, Sveen TH. Prevalence of psychiatric disorders in preschoolers. *Journal of Child Psychology and Psychiatry*. 2012;53(6):695–705.
9. Egger HL, Angold A. Common emotional and behavioral disorders in preschool children: Presentation, nosology, and epidemiology. *Journal of Child Psychology and Psychiatry*. 2006;47(3–4):313–337.
10. Finsaas MC, Bufferd SJ, Dougherty LR, Carlson GA, Klein DN. Preschool psychiatric disorders: Homotypic and heterotypic continuity through middle childhood and early adolescence. *Psychological Medicine*. 2018;48(13):2159–2168.
11. Copeland WE, Wolke D, Shanahan L, Costello J. Adult functional outcomes of common childhood psychiatric problems: A prospective, longitudinal study. *JAMA Psychiatry*. 2015;72(9):892–899.
12. Shanahan L, Zucker N, Copeland WE, Bondy CL, Egger HL, Costello EJ. Childhood somatic complaints predict generalized anxiety and depressive disorders during young adulthood in a community sample. *Psychological Medicine*. 2015;45(8):1721–1730.

13. Keenan K, Wakschlag LS. Can a valid diagnosis of disruptive behavior disorder be made in preschool children? *American Journal of Psychiatry.* 2002;159(3):351–358.

14. Lahey BB, Lee SS, Sibley MH, Applegate B, Molina BSG, Pelham WE. Predictors of adolescent outcomes among 4–6 year old children with attention-deficit/hyperactivity disorder. *Journal of Abnormal Psychology.* 2016;125:168–181.

15. Demmer DH, Hooley M, Sheen J, McGillivray JA, Lum JAG. Sex differences in the prevalence of oppositional defiant disorder during middle childhood: A meta-analysis. *Journal of Abnormal Child Psychology.* 2017;45(2):313–325.

16. Hart EL, Lahey BB, Loeber R, Applegate B, Green SM, Frick PJ. Developmental change in attention-deficit hyperactivity disorder in boys: A four-year longitudinal study. *Journal of Abnormal Child Psychology.* 1995;23:729–749.

17. Husby SM, Wichstrom L. Interrelationships and continuities in symptoms of oppositional defiant and conduct disorders from age 4 to 10 in the community. *Journal of Abnormal Child Psychology.* 2017;45(5):947–958.

18. Lahey BB, Van Hulle CA, Rathouz PJ, Rodgers JL, D'Onofrio BM, Waldman ID. Are oppositional-defiant and hyperactive-inattentive symptoms developmental precursors to conduct problems in late childhood? Genetic and environmental links. *Journal of Abnormal Child Psychology.* 2009;37:45–58.

19. Burke JD, Waldman I, Lahey BB. Predictive validity of childhood oppositional defiant disorder and conduct disorder: Implications for the DSM-V. *Journal of Abnormal Psychology.* 2010;119(4):739–751.

20. Lahey BB, Schwab-Stone M, Goodman SH, et al. Age and gender differences in oppositional behavior and conduct problems: A cross-sectional household study of middle childhood and adolescence. *Journal of Abnormal Psychology.* 2000;109(3):488–503.

21. Gutman LM, Joshi H, Parsonage M, Schoon I. Gender-specific trajectories of conduct problems from ages 3 to 11. *Journal of Abnormal Child Psychology.* 2018;46(7):1467–1480.

22. Lahey BB, Schwab-Stone M, Goodman SH, et al. Age and gender differences in oppositional behavior and conduct problems: A cross-sectional household study of middle childhood and adolescence. *Journal of Abnormal Psychology.* 2000;109:488–503.

23. Lahey BB, Van Hulle CA, Waldman ID, et al. Testing descriptive hypotheses regarding sex differences in the development of conduct problems and delinquency. *Journal of Abnormal Child Psychology.* 2006;34:737–755.

24. Loeber R, Green SM, Keenan K, Lahey BB. Which boys will fare worse? Early predictors of the onset of conduct disorder in a six-year longitudinal study. *Journal of the American Academy of Child and Adolescent Psychiatry.* 1995;34:499–509.

25. Wertz J, Agnew-Blais J, Caspi A, et al. From childhood conduct problems to poor functioning at age 18 years: Examining explanations in a longitudinal cohort study. *Journal of the American Academy of Child and Adolescent Psychiatry.* 2018;57(1):54–60.

26. Bufferd SJ, Dougherty LR, Carlson GA, Rose S, Klein DN. Psychiatric disorders in preschoolers: Continuity from ages 3 to 6. *American Journal of Psychiatry.* 2012;169:1157–1164.

27. Franz L, Angold A, Copeland W, Costello EJ, Towe-Goodman N, Egger H. Preschool anxiety disorders in pediatric primary care: Prevalence and comorbidity. *Journal of the American Academy of Child and Adolescent Psychiatry.* 2013;52(12):1294–1303.

28. ten Berge M, Veerkamp JSJ, Hoogstraten J, Prins PJM. Childhood dental fear in the Netherlands: Prevalence and normative data. *Community Dentistry and Oral Epidemiology.* 2002;30(2):101–107.

29. Lichtenstein P, Annas P. Heritability and prevalence of specific fears and phobias in childhood. *Journal of Child Psychology and Psychiatry.* 2000;41(7):927–937.

30. Ollendick TH, King NJ, Frary RB. Fears in children and adolescents: Reliability and generalizability across gender, age, and nationality. *Behaviour Research and Therapy.* 1989;27(1):19–26.

31. Bowen RC, Offord DR, Boyle MH. The prevalence of overanxious disorder and separation disorder: Result from the Ontario Child Health Study. *Journal of the American Academy of Child and Adolescent Psychiatry.* 1990;29(5):753–758.

32. Muris P, Merckelbach H, Schmidt T, Mayer B. The revised version of the Screen for Child Anxiety Related Emotional Disorders (SCARED-R): Factor structure in normal children. *Personality and Individual Differences.* 1999;26(1):99–112.

33. King NJ, Gullone E, Ollendick TH. Manifest anxiety and fearfulness in children and adolescents. *Journal of Genetic Psychology.* 1992;153(1):63–73.

34. Copeland WE, Angold A, Shanahan L, Costello EJ. Longitudinal patterns of anxiety from childhood to adulthood: The Great Smoky Mountains Study. *Journal of the American Academy of Child and Adolescent Psychiatry.* 2014;53(1):21–33.

35. Gullone E, King NJ. Three-year follow-up of normal fear in children and adolescents aged 7 to 18 years. *British Journal of Developmental Psychology.* 1997;15:97–111.

36. Costello EJ, Copeland W, Angold A. Trends in psychopathology across the adolescent years: What changes when children become adolescents, and when adolescents become adults? *Journal of Child Psychology and Psychiatry.* 2011;52:1015–1025.

37. Kim SJ, Kim BN, Cho SC, et al. The prevalence of specific phobia and associated co-morbid features in children and adolescents. *Journal of Anxiety Disorders.* 2010;24(6):629–634.

38. Baghdadli A, Michelon C, Pernon E, et al. Adaptive trajectories and early risk factors in the autism spectrum: A 15-year prospective study. *Autism Research.* 2018;11(11):1455–1467.

39. Copeland WE, Shanahan L, Costello EJ, Angold A. Childhood and adolescent psychiatric disorders as predictors of young adult disorders. *Archives of General Psychiatry.* 2009;66(7):764–772.

40. Copeland WE, Adair CE, Smetanin P, et al. Diagnostic transitions from childhood to adolescence to early adulthood. *Journal of Child Psychology and Psychiatry.* 2013;54:791–799.

41. Newman DL, Moffitt TE, Caspi A, Magdol L, Silva PA, Stanton WR. Psychiatric disorder in a birth cohort of young adults: Prevalence, comorbidity, clinical significance, and new case incidence from ages 11 to 21. *Journal of Consulting and Clinical Psychology.* 1996;64(3):552–562.

42. Costello EJ, Maughan B. Annual research review: Optimal outcomes of child and adolescent mental illness. *Journal of Child Psychology and Psychiatry.* 2015;56(3):324–341.

43. Steinhausen HC, Jakobsen H. Incidence rates of treated mental disorders in childhood and adolescence in a complete nationwide birth cohort. *Journal of Clinical Psychiatry.* 2019;80(3):17m12012.

44. Pedersen CB, Mors O, Bertelsen A, et al. A comprehensive nationwide study of the incidence rate and lifetime risk for treated mental disorders. *JAMA Psychiatry.* 2014;71(5):573–581.

45. Abecasis GR, Cardon LR, Cookson WOC. A general test of association for quantitative traits in nuclear families. *American Journal of Human Genetics.* 2000;66:279–292.

46. Wittchen HU, Fehm L. Epidemiology and natural course of social fears and social phobia. *Acta Psychiatrica Scandinavica.* 2003;108:4–18.

47. Gren-Landell M, Tillfors M, Furmark T, Bohlin G, Andersson G, Svedin CG. Social phobia in Swedish adolescents: Prevalence and gender differences. *Social Psychiatry and Psychiatric Epidemiology.* 2009;44(1):1–7.

48. Seedat S, Scott KM, Angermeyer MC, et al. Cross-national associations between gender and mental disorders in the World Health Organization World Mental Health Surveys. *Archives of General Psychiatry.* 2009;66:785–795.

49. Rao PA, Beidel DC, Turner SM, Ammerman RT, Crosby LE, Sallee FR. Social anxiety disorder in childhood and adolescence: Descriptive psychopathology. *Behaviour Research and Therapy.* 2007;45(6):1181–1191.

50. Costello EJ, Egger HL, Angold A. The developmental epidemiology of anxiety disorders: Phenomenology, prevalence, and comorbidity. *Child and Adolescent Psychiatric Clinics of North America.* 2005;14(4):631–648.

51. Hasin DS, Grant BF. The National Epidemiologic Survey on Alcohol and Related Conditions (NESARC) Waves 1 and 2: Review and

summary of findings. *Social Psychiatry and Psychiatric Epidemiology.* 2015;50(11):1609–1640.

52. Kossowsky J, Pfaltz MC, Schneider S, Taeymans J, Locher C, Gaab J. The separation anxiety hypothesis of panic disorder revisited: A meta-analysis. *American Journal of Psychiatry.* 2013;170(7):768–781.

53. Roberson-Nay R, Eaves LJ, Hettema JM, Kendler KS, Silberg JL. Childhood separation anxiety and adult onset panic attacks share a common genetic diathesis. *Depression and Anxiety.* 2012;29(4):320–327.

54. Copeland WE, Shanahan L, Costello EJ, Angold A. Childhood and adolescent psychiatric disorders as predictors of young adult disorders. *Archives of General Psychiatry.* 2009;66:764–772.

55. Klein DN, Glenn CR, Kosty DB, Seeley JR, Rohde P, Lewinsohn PM. Predictors of first lifetime onset of major depressive disorder in young adulthood. *Journal of Abnormal Psychology.* 2013;122(1):1–6.

56. Sentse M, Kretschmer T, de Haan A, Prinzie P. Conduct problem trajectories between age 4 and 17 and their association with behavioral adjustment in emerging adulthood. *Journal of Youth and Adolescence.* 2017;46(8):1633–1642.

57. Loeber R, Menting B, Lynam DR, et al. Findings from the Pittsburgh Youth Study: Cognitive impulsivity and intelligence as predictors of the age–crime curve. *Journal of the American Academy of Child and Adolescent Psychiatry.* 2012;51:1136–1149.

58. Rivenbark JG, Odgers CL, Caspi A, et al. The high societal costs of childhood conduct problems: Evidence from administrative records up to age 38 in a longitudinal birth cohort. *Journal of Child Psychology and Psychiatry.* 2018;59(6):703–710.

59. Falk O, Wallinius M, Lundstrom S, Frisell T, Anckarsater H, Kerekes N. The 1% of the population accountable for 63% of all violent crime convictions. *Social Psychiatry and Psychiatric Epidemiology.* 2014;49(4):559–571.

60. Eaton NR, Keyes KM, Krueger RF, et al. An invariant dimensional liability model of gender differences in mental disorder prevalence: Evidence from a national sample. *Journal of Abnormal Psychology.* 2012;121:282–288.

61. Robins LN. Conduct disorder. *Journal of Child Psychology and Psychiatry.* 1991;32:193–212.

62. Chen P, Jacobson KC. Developmental trajectories of substance use from early adolescence to young adulthood: Gender and racial/ethnic differences. *Journal of Adolescent Health.* 2012;50(2):154–163.

63. McHugh RK, Votaw VR, Sugarman DE, Greenfield SF. Sex and gender differences in substance use disorders. *Clinical Psychology Review.* 2018;66:12–23.

64. Pingault JB, Cote SM, Galera C, et al. Childhood trajectories of inattention, hyperactivity and oppositional behaviors and prediction of substance abuse/dependence: A 15-year longitudinal population-based study. *Molecular Psychiatry.* 2013;18(7):806–812.

65. Knop J, Penick EC, Nickel EJ, et al. Childhood ADHD and conduct disorder as independent predictors of male alcohol dependence at age 40. *Journal of Studies on Alcohol and Drugs.* 2009;70(2):169–177.

66. Heron J, Barker ED, Joinson C, et al. Childhood conduct disorder trajectories, prior risk factors and cannabis use at age 16: Birth cohort study. *Addiction.* 2013;108(12):2129–2138.

67. Hafner H, Maurer K, Loffler W, et al. The epidemiology of early schizophrenia: Influence of age and gender on onset and early course. *British Journal of Psychiatry.* 1994;164:29–38.

68. Ferrari AJ, Stockings E, Khoo JP, et al. The prevalence and burden of bipolar disorder: Findings from the Global Burden of Disease Study 2013. *Bipolar Disorders.* 2016;18(5):440–450.

69. Kennedy N, Everitt B, Boydell J, Van Os J, Jones PB, Murray RM. Incidence and distribution of first-episode mania by age: Results from a 35-year study. *Psychological Medicine.* 2005;35(6):855–863.

70. Kennedy N, Boydell J, Kalidindi S, et al. Gender differences in incidence and age at onset of mania and bipolar disorder over a 35-year period in Camberwell, England. *American Journal of Psychiatry.* 2005;162(2):257–262.

71. Kessler RC, Birnbaum HG, Shahly V, et al. Age differences in the prevalence and co-morbidity of DSM-IV major depressive episodes: Results from the WHO World Mental Health Survey Initiative. *Depression and Anxiety.* 2010;27:351–364.

72. Salk RH, Hyde JS, Abramson LY. Gender differences in depression in representative national samples: Meta-analyses of diagnoses and symptoms. *Psychological Bulletin.* 2017;143(8):783–822.

73. Lewinsohn PM, Duncan EM, Stanton AK, Hautzinger M. Age at 1st onset for nonbipolar depression. *Journal of Abnormal Psychology.* 1986;95(4):378–383.

74. Newman SC, Bland RC. Incidence of mental disorders in Edmonton: Estimates of rates and methodological issues. *Journal of Psychiatric Research.* 1998;32(5):273–282.

75. Rorsman B, Grasbeck A, Hagnell O, et al. A prospective study of 1st-incidence depression: The Lundby Study, 1957–72. *British Journal of Psychiatry.* 1990;156:336–342.

76. Swahn MH, Bossarte RM. Gender, early alcohol use, and suicide ideation and attempts: Findings from the 2005 Youth Risk Behavior Survey. *Journal of Adolescent Health.* 2007;41(2):175–181.

77. Zhang J, McKeown RE, Hussey JR, Thompson SJ, Woods JR. Gender differences in risk factors for attempted suicide among young adults: Findings from the Third National Health and Nutrition Examination Survey. *Annals of Epidemiology.* 2005;15(2):167–174.

78. Pickles A, Aglan A, Collishaw S, Messer J, Rutter M, Maughan B. Predictors of suicidality across the life span: The Isle of Wight study. *Psychological Medicine*. 2010;40(9):1453–1466.

79. Choo CC, Harris KM, Ho RC. Prediction of lethality in suicide attempts: Gender matters. *Omega*. 2019;80(1):87–103.

80. Carstensen LL, Shavit YZ, Barnes JT. Age advantages in emotional experience persist even under threat from the COVID-19 pandemic. *Psychological Science*. 2020;31:1374–1385.

81. Goldstein RB, Chou SP, Saha TD, et al. The epidemiology of antisocial behavioral syndromes in adulthood: Results from the National Epidemiologic Survey on Alcohol and Related Conditions–III. *Journal of Clinical Psychiatry*. 2017;78(1):90–98.

82. Goldstein RB, Grant BF. Three-year follow-up of syndromal antisocial behavior in adults: Results from the Wave 2 National Epidemiologic Survey on Alcohol and Related Conditions. *Journal of Clinical Psychiatry*. 2009;70(9):1237–1249.

83. Hoertel N, McMahon K, Olfson M, et al. A dimensional liability model of age differences in mental disorder prevalence: Evidence from a national sample. *Journal of Psychiatric Research*. 2015;64:107–113.

84. Grant BF, Goldstein RB, Saha TD, et al. Epidemiology of DSM-5 alcohol use disorder: Results from the National Epidemiologic Survey on Alcohol and Related Conditions III. *JAMA Psychiatry*. 2015;72(8):757–766.

85. Moffitt TE, Caspi A, Taylor A, et al. How common are common mental disorders? Evidence that lifetime prevalence rates are doubled by prospective versus retrospective ascertainment. *Psychological Medicine*. 2010;40:899–909.

86. Schaefer JD, Caspi A, Belsky DW, et al. Enduring mental health: Prevalence and prediction. *Journal of Abnormal Psychology*. 2017;126(2):212–224.

87. Lahey BB, Zald DH, Hakes JK, Krueger RF, Rathouz PJ. Patterns of heterotypic continuity associated with the cross-sectional correlational structure of prevalent mental disorders in adults. *JAMA Psychiatry*. 2014;71:989–996.

88. Blanco C, Wall MM, Wang S, Olfson M. Examining heterotypic continuity of psychopathology: A prospective national study. *Psychological Medicine*. 2017;47(12):2097–2106.

89. Plana-Ripoll O, Pedersen CB, Holtz Y, et al. Exploring comorbidity within mental disorders among a Danish national population. *JAMA Psychiatry*. 2019;76(3):259–270.

90. Lahey BB, Loeber R, Burke J, Rathouz PJ, McBurnett K. Waxing and waning in concert: Dynamic comorbidity of conduct disorder with other disruptive and emotional problems over 17 years among clinic-referred boys. *Journal of Abnormal Psychology*. 2002;111:556–567.

91. Costello EJ, Mustillo S, Erkanli A, Keeler G, Angold A. Prevalence and development of psychiatric disorders in childhood and adolescence. *Archives of General Psychiatry*. 2003;60:837–844.

92. Moffitt TE, Harrington H, Caspi A, et al. Depression and generalized anxiety disorder: Cumulative and sequential comorbidity in a birth cohort followed prospectively to age 32 years. *Archives of General Psychiatry*. 2007;64:651–660.

93. Halperin JM, Schulz KP. Revisiting the role of the prefrontal cortex in the pathophysiology of attention-deficit/hyperactivity disorder. *Psychological Bulletin*. 2006;132:560–581.

94. Hart H, Radua J, Nakao T, Mataix-Cols D, Rubia K. Meta-analysis of functional magnetic resonance imaging studies of inhibition and attention in attention-deficit/hyperactivity disorder exploring task-specific, stimulant medication, and age effects. *JAMA Psychiatry*. 2013;70(2):185–198.

95. Hoogman M, Bralten J, Hibar DP, et al. Subcortical brain volume differences in participants with attention deficit hyperactivity disorder in children and adults: A cross-sectional mega-analysis. *Lancet Psychiatry*. 2017;4(4):310–319.

96. Paus T, Keshavan M, Giedd JN. Why do many psychiatric disorders emerge during adolescence? *Nature Reviews Neuroscience*. 2008;9(12):947–957.

97. Cox KH, Bonthuis PJ, Rissman EF. Mouse model systems to study sex chromosome genes and behavior: Relevance to humans. *Frontiers in Neuroendocrinology*. 2014;35(4):405–419.

98. Abel KM, Drake R, Goldstein JM. Sex differences in schizophrenia. *International Review of Psychiatry*. 2010;22(5):417–428.

99. Ngun TC, Ghahramani N, Sanchez FJ, Bocklandt S, Vilain E. The genetics of sex differences in brain and behavior. *Frontiers in Neuroendocrinology*. 2011;32(2):227–246.

100. Rutter M, Caspi A, Moffitt TE. Using sex differences in psychopathology to study causal mechanisms: Unifying issues and research strategies. *Journal of Child Psychology and Psychiatry*. 2003;44(8):1092–1115.

101. Parsch J, Ellegren H. The evolutionary causes and consequences of sex-biased gene expression. *Nature Reviews Genetics*. 2013;14(2):83–87.

102. Trabzuni D, Ramasamy A, Imran S, et al. Widespread sex differences in gene expression and splicing in the adult human brain. *Nature Communications*. 2013;4:2771.

103. Kuehner C. Why is depression more common among women than among men? *Lancet Psychiatry*. 2017;4(2):146–158.

104. Torre M. Attrition from male-dominated occupations: Variation among occupations and women. *Sociological Perspectives*. 2017;60(4):665–684.

105. Iverson KM, Dick A, McLaughlin KA, et al. Exposure to interpersonal violence and its associations with psychiatric morbidity in a US national sample: A gender comparison. *Psychology of Violence*. 2013;3(3):273–287.

106. Bebbington PE, Cooper C, Minot S, et al. Suicide attempts, gender, and sexual abuse: Data from the 2000 British Psychiatric Morbidity Survey. *American Journal of Psychiatry.* 2009;166(10):1135–1140.

107. Lavoie L, Dupere V, Dion E, Crosnoe R, Lacourse E, Archambault I. Gender differences in adolescents' exposure to stressful life events and differential links to impaired school functioning. *Journal of Abnormal Child Psychology.* 2019;47(6):1053–1064.

108. Antecol H, Barcus VE, Cobb-Clark D. Gender-biased behavior at work: Exploring the relationship between sexual harassment and sex discrimination. *Journal of Economic Psychology.* 2009;30(5):782–792.

109. Bugge I, Dyb G, Stensland SO, Ekeberg O, Wentzel-Larsen T, Diseth TH. Physical injury and posttraumatic stress reactions: A study of the survivors of the 2011 shooting massacre on Utoya Island, Norway. *Journal of Psychosomatic Research.* 2015;79(5):384–390.

110. Cloninger CR, Christiansen KO, Reich T, Gottesman II. Implications of sex differences in the prevalences of antisocial personality, alcoholism, and criminality for familial transmission. *Archives of General Psychiatry.* 1978;35:941–951.

111. Taylor MJ, Lichtenstein P, Larsson H, Anckarsater H, Greven CU, Ronald A. Is there a female protective effect against attention-deficit/hyperactivity disorder? Evidence from two representative twin samples. *Journal of the American Academy of Child and Adolescent Psychiatry.* 2016;55(6):504–512.

112. Robinson EB, Lichtenstein P, Anckarsater H, Happe F, Ronald A. Examining and interpreting the female protective effect against autistic behavior. *Proceedings of the National Academy of Sciences of the United States of America.* 2013;110(13):5258–5262.

113. Van Hulle CA, Rodgers JL, D'Onofrio BM, Waldman ID, Lahey BB. Sex differences in the causes of self-reported adolescent delinquency. *Journal of Abnormal Psychology.* 2007;116(2):236–248.

8

Ordinary Origins of Psychological Problems

Genetic–Environmental Interplay

We will understand psychological problems much better when we understand their causes. Why do some people have psychological problems and others do not? Why do different people have different problems? These are complicated and challenging questions, but I am going to present *tentative* answers based on what is known to date. These statements should be viewed only as strong hypotheses rather than conclusions. The ratio of what we know to what we do not know is still pretty poor. Nonetheless, I summarize both basic facts and the results of exciting recent research on the causes of psychological problems in this and Chapter 9.

I first focus on insights learned from studies of the genetic and environmental influences on psychological problems. In this discussion, I never assert that a dimension of psychological problems is caused by our genes or caused by our environments (i.e., our experiences). The focus is always on how both genetics and environments work together to influence psychological problems. Keep in mind that genes and environments work in the same ordinary ways to influence the entire spectrum of behavior, from highly adaptive to highly problematic. As I keep saying, psychological problems arise in ordinary ways.

Basic Gene Biology and Inheritance

To be sure that we are all starting this discussion from the same point, I begin with a primer on the biological bases of inheritance. Some readers with a solid knowledge of genetics will want to skim or skip this section. In the nuclei of all of the cells in our bodies, there are two-sided strands of deoxyribonucleic acid (DNA) twisted into the shape of a double helix that can be said to carry the code of inheritance. Between the two strands are pairs of complex molecules called *nucleotides*. There are four different nucleotides, which are often referred to by their first letters: adenine (A), cytosine (C), guanine (G), and thymine (T). Some segments of DNA are termed *genes* because they contain the code for the synthesis of one of the proteins that make up our bodies, including proteins in the brain and neuroendocrine systems that are intimately linked to our behavior. The sequence of letters—nucleotides—in our DNA determines the protein that will be synthesized when the gene is set into motion by other substances, called transcription factors. We have almost 3 billion nucleotides and more than 20,000 genes that code for proteins.

The strands of DNA are coiled and wrapped many times on themselves to form structures called *chromosomes*. In the cells of humans, there are 23 pairs of chromosomes. Each chromosome contains many different genes. The vast majority of human genes do not vary from individual to individual—they make all human beings similar enough to distinguish us from dogs, lizards, and cabbages. Nonetheless, there is an important minority of genes that exist in multiple forms in the population, referred to as *polymorphic genes*. Each version of a polymorphic gene is called an *allele*. Crucially, these different alleles control the differences in protein synthesis that contribute to differences among human beings in everything from eye color and height to our psychological characteristics. When the pair of two alleles of polymorphic genes inherited from the parents is considered together, the pair is termed a *genotype*. This is in contrast to the term *phenotype*, which refers to the trait we are considering: height, intelligence, or in our case, dimensions of psychological problems.

If you care about psychological problems and think science can shed light on them, the fact that larger and better studies have been conducted every year since the human genome was sequenced of associations between genotypes and behavioral phenotypes is incredibly exciting. These studies of tens of thousands of people have mostly used a research tool based on the fact that some polymorphic alleles differ by only a single letter (i.e., one nucleotide) in the DNA sequence of the gene—referred to as *single nucleotide polymorphisms* (SNPs). Other variations in alleles of genes that are more complex, involving such things as different numbers of repeats of a sequence of letters, also are important, but SNPs have been studied extensively in recent years both for the good reason that they are informative and for the bad reason that they can be studied at the molecular level more cheaply than other polymorphisms. The best science is expensive and we do not invest enough in it, but we have already learned a lot on a tight budget.

Heritability

Much of what we currently know about the interplay of genetic and environmental influences on psychological problems was learned before we could measure variations in genetic sequences at the molecular level. The original methods of estimating the importance of genetic influences in the interplay with experiences that influence our psychological functioning made use of two kinds of "experiments of nature" without measuring genes at the molecular level: studies of twins and studies of adopted children.

I briefly described the logic of twin studies in Chapter 5, but I expand on it here. All persons, whether a twin or not, randomly receive one allele of each polymorphic gene from each of our two biological parents. As a result of this random process, full siblings with the same two biological parents tend to resemble one another physically and psychologically to a considerable degree because, on average, full siblings share 50% of their alleles of polymorphic genes.

It gets really interesting when we look at this process in the two different kinds of twins. One kind of twins results from two male sperm independently fertilizing two separate female eggs. If both fertilized eggs—now called zygotes—implant in the uterus and grow to birth, the result is a pair of dizygotic or paternal twins. They are not identical twins because they arose from two different eggs and two different sperm cells. As a result, they share 50% of their alleles of polymorphic genes on average, just like full siblings, because that is what dizygotic twins are in genetic terms—two full siblings, who just happened to be in the womb and born at the same time.

The other kind of twins arises from one zygote created by the fertilization of one egg by one sperm. These twins are called monozygotic, maternal, or identical twins. In this case, the zygote splits during the early stages of growth and each part implants in the uterus separately and grows to birth. Because the single zygote that splits is the result of the union of just one egg and one sperm, both twins have the same DNA sequence and hence the same genes. A lot can happen to make monozygotic differences different over time, including changes in how their genes are expressed, but we can use the differences between monozygotic and dizygotic twins in their DNA sequences to draw inferences about the role of genes and environments in psychological functioning. These inferences are based on several assumptions, so the fact that many of the conclusions from twin studies have been confirmed using other methods of study makes us more confident in them.

We can draw inferences about genetic and environmental influences on a phenotype from twin studies as follows: Because both monozygotic and dizygotic twins were in the womb at the same time, were raised in the same families who lived in the same neighborhoods, and so on, we can assume that they do not differ in the basic aspects of their environments that are shared by family members. They can differ in the specific experiences that each twin has (e.g., if one is mugged and the other is not), but they cannot differ in the things that twins automatically share in common (e.g., the ages of their parents, the fact that the family was evicted from their home when the twins were age 3 years and were homeless for 6 months, and so on).

Thus, both monozygotic and dizygotic twin pairs share their environments to a great extent. The difference is that monozygotic twins share 100% of their polymorphic genes and dizygotic twins only share 50% of them. So, if we ask both members of both kinds of twin pairs to complete a measure of, for example, psychotic experiences and we find that the pairs of monozygotic twins are more similar to one another on this measure than are pairs of dizygotic twins, we can *infer* that genes are one of the factors that influence psychotic behavior. This is because the only way in which monozygotic twin pairs are more similar to one another than are dizygotic twin pairs is the much greater degree of similarity in the DNA sequences in monozygotic twin pairs. We can even use the magnitude of the difference in the correlations between monozygotic and dizygotic twin pairs on any dimension of behavior to mathematically estimate the proportion of differences on the dimension among people in the population that is attributable to genetic factors. This estimate is referred to as the *heritability* of the phenotype.

Different dimensions of psychological problems have different degrees of heritability that give us one indication of the role of genes in their origins. For example, twin studies have estimated the heritability of autism spectrum disorder to be at least 80%,[1] meaning that 80% of the differences among people in their autistic problems that are serious enough to meet *Diagnostic and Statistical Manual of Mental Disorders* (DSM) criteria for the diagnosis of autism spectrum disorder are due to genetic differences among people. As discussed later, this does not mean that the environment plays no role in the origins of autistic problems—it most certainly does—but it means that genetic influences on autism spectrum problems are very important in the origins of these problems. Twin studies also estimate the heritability of schizophrenia[2] and attention-deficit/hyperactivity disorder problems[3,4] to be about 80%, but not all dimensions of psychological problems have such high heritabilities. The heritability estimate for alcohol dependence is 60%,[5] and estimates of the heritability of problems of fear, anxiety, and depression range from 30% to 50%.[6-8]

To avoid a misunderstanding of the concept of heritability, we should look more closely at schizophrenia as an example. This discussion also will help readers avoid misunderstanding their personal risk for developing schizophrenia if they have a biological relative who has been given this diagnosis. We use the fact that about 1% of the population meets DSM criteria for schizophrenia in any year as the "base rate" of schizophrenia to help us think quantitatively about the role of genes in schizophrenia. People with a dizygotic twin, a full sibling, or a biological parent with the diagnosis of schizophrenia—which are all biological relatives that share an average of 50% of their polymorphic genes—have only about a 10% chance of meeting criteria for schizophrenia.[9] Even persons with a monozygotic twin who has been given the diagnosis of schizophrenia—with whom they share 100% of their DNA sequence—have only about a 50% chance of being given the diagnosis of schizophrenia at some time during their lives.[9] This shows that genes are certainly not the only factors that influence risk for schizophrenic problems. Nonetheless, the heritability of the diagnosis of schizophrenia is correctly estimated to be very high because the chances that a person with a monozygotic twin with schizophrenia will be given that diagnosis are 50 times higher than the base rate of 1% in the general population, whereas the chances for a dizygotic twin of someone with a diagnosis of schizophrenia—who shares 50% of their DNA sequences on average—are 10 times greater than the risk for a random person in the population. These facts reveal the strong role played by genetics but make it clear that the environment also plays an important role. If that were not the case, monozygotic twins would completely resemble each other on schizophrenic problems. Not even people with exactly the same DNA sequence will always have the same psychological problems. Genes are important, but they certainly do not dictate our psychological destinies.

When the human genome was first sequenced, the high heritability estimates for some kinds of psychological problems in twin studies launched many studies that fully expected to find the polymorphic genes that increased risk for each mental disorder at the molecular level. The first generation of such studies failed to find genes for any dimension of psychological problems, but they taught us some important lessons. Most important, these first studies taught us that there is no dimension of psychological problems for which the genetic risk is encoded by a single polymorphic gene. Some physical diseases are linked to a single gene, such as sickle cell anemia and cystic fibrosis, but dimensions of psychological problems are *polygenic*. This means that hundreds or thousands of variations in DNA contribute to the net genetic risk for each kind of psychological problem. Each of these many genetic polymorphisms accounts for only a tiny amount of the heritability of each psychological problem individually, so a method of combining them to understand their substantial joint effect was needed.

Consequently, *polygenic risk scores* were developed that combine information from variations in large numbers of SNPs to quantify the genetic influences on each dimension of psychological problems. The polygenic risk score is a weighted combination of many SNPs, with the weight of each SNP based on its strength of association with the dimension estimated in a large reference sample.[10] Polygenic risk scores do not capture all of the heritability encoded in our DNA sequences because SNPs are only one kind of variation in DNA sequences, and there is still a tremendous amount to learn about how all forms of variations in DNA jointly contribute to the genetic risk for psychological problems.[11] Nonetheless, polygenic risk scores generally confirm much of what has been learned from twin studies about genetic risk for many traits.[12] We now have strong evidence that variation in DNA sequences is one of the factors that creates risk for all kinds of psychological problems, often to considerable extents.

Pleiotropy and Correlated Dimensions of Psychological Problems

One of the themes of this book, which you have heard many times before, is that all dimensions of psychological problems are positively correlated with one another. As detailed in Chapter 6, all dimensions are correlated strongly enough that we can hypothesize a general factor of psychological problems that reflects those robust and widespread correlations. In addition, several smaller groups of dimensions of psychological problems are more highly correlated with one another than with dimensions in other small groups. For example, internalizing dimensions are more correlated with one another than they are with externalizing or psychotic dimensions. Beginning with a paper in 2011, my colleagues and I hypothesized that this hierarchical structure is mostly caused by the operation of more than one set of highly nonspecific (or pleiotropic) genes.[13] *Pleiotropy* means that each polymorphic gene influences more than one phenotype. Considered together, many studies[14] now suggest that many genetic factors are broadly pleiotropic—directly or indirectly influencing all dimensions of psychological problems through the general factor—whereas other sets of genetic factors are more narrowly pleiotropic, influencing all dimensions within a single domain, such as all externalizing dimensions, but not influencing dimensions in other domains. Although each dimension of psychological problems also is influenced by genetic influences that are specific to only that dimension, the nonspecific or pleiotropic genetic influences that are shared by multiple dimensions of psychological problems cause all dimensions to be correlated. As stated in Chapter 7, this suggests that many nonspecific genetic factors influence the likelihood of a person having *some kind* of psychological problems but *not which kind* of problems.[13,14]

That was a radical departure from thinking that each categorical mental disorder is associated with its own genes, which was the model that guided our thinking until very recently, but a growing number of scientists now share this view.[15-17] The notion that pleiotropic genes play a prominent role in psychological problems has also been supported in very large-scale studies using molecular measurement. Polygenic risk scores based on SNPs reveal that some sets of alleles are pleiotropically associated with multiple kinds of psychological problems, whereas other alleles are specific to only one dimension.[15-17] To be sure, there is still a lot to be learned, but it appears that one reason that all dimensions of psychological problems are correlated is the pleiotropic nature of many genes.

Interplay of Genes and Environments

No dimension of psychological problems can ever be said to be influenced only by genes or only by environments; it is always both. Psychological problems are the result of both nature and nurture. One of the most important things we have learned in the past 30 years is that genetic and environmental influences on psychological problems work together in a fascinatingly complex interplay. Perhaps the most important paper written on genes and environments since Darwin and Mendel was the astute and cogent framing of gene–environment interplay by Robert Plomin, John DeFries, and John Loehlin.[18] It is must reading for serious students of human behavior. They posited that genes and environments influence our adaptive and maladaptive behavior through gene–environment correlations and gene–environment interactions, which are defined and discussed next.

Gene–Environment Correlations

We naturally think of the genes inside our cells and the environments in which we live as two separate things, but in an extremely important way, they are not! Our environmental risks for any trait are not independent of our genetic risks. This is an amazingly important insight.[18] Our genes and environments often become correlated with one another so that persons who are genetically influenced to have high levels of psychological problems also wind up in social environments that promote the same psychological problems. These gene–environment correlations arise in three different ways:

- *Passive gene–environment correlation*: Genes and environments become correlated simply because parents both pass genes to their children and provide environments for their children that are related to those genes. To take a positive example, the genes of intelligent parents are passed to their children and influence their children's intelligence. In addition, intelligent parents tend to provide intellectually stimulating child-rearing environments for their children. Therefore, the children's genes relevant to intelligence are correlated with their stimulating child-rearing environments. The same thing happens with parents who tend to be depressed partly for genetic reasons. They may both provide an emotionally cold child-rearing environment at times and pass on their risk genotypes for depression to their children. Thus, the child's risk for depression is increased due to both their child-rearing environment and their correlated genes. This kind of "double whammy" of correlated risk genes and risk environments is said to arise passively because it is not dependent on the child's behavior, unlike the next two ways in which genes and environments become correlated.
- *Evocative gene–environment correlation*: The varying genotypes in people often become correlated with our environments because they influence the environments in which we live. To a very real extent, we create worlds that reflect our genes! When children inherit genetic variants that promote their being irritable, defiant, and reactively aggressive, for example, they behave in ways that often evoke criticism and punishment for their behavior from

their parents and teachers and also evoke fractious interactions with peers. Their risk genes and risk environments become correlated because of their genetically influenced behavior. Thus, children who are genetically predisposed to irritable and aggressive behavior are likely to live in a critical and rejecting social world that is partly of their own creation, which makes their maladaptive behavior that much worse. This does not only occur in childhood, of course. Chronically irritable and aggressive adults are not fun to be around, and their behavior shapes their social environments. Similarly, every genetically influenced dimension of psychological problems—they are all influenced by genetic variations to some extent—can evoke responses from other people that influence their social environments, which often make their problems worse. Thus, evocative gene–environment correlations arise when genetically influenced characteristics of persons evoke changes in their environments, causing risk genes to be correlated with risk environments.

- *Selective gene-environment correlation*: Genes and environments also can become correlated because the genetically influenced characteristics of individuals influence their environments in another way that is subtly different from evocative gene–environment correlations. Often, genetically influenced characteristics lead persons to "select" environments that match those characteristics. This is usually not a conscious process of selection, as in selecting a brand of toothpaste. For example, the genetic variants of some persons may promote a schizoid-like discomfort in being with other people, which may mean that living at home with relatives and holding most jobs are so uncomfortable that these individuals wind up living on the streets. This correlates their genetic risk for schizoid behavior with the adverse environment of the street. Everything from genetically influenced social dependence to agoraphobic anxiety and psychotic behavior selects people into certain environments rather than others in similar ways.

Thus, one way in which genes and environments work together is by becoming correlated with one another through the three types of gene–environment correlation. They "gang up" on the individual. People with genetic dispositions to alcohol abuse and dependence are more likely to have been raised by parents who did not use alcohol adaptively, to evoke stressful interactions with others that lead to moods that are "medicated" by alcohol, and to have few friends other than drinking buddies who promote drinking.

Another way of saying what gene–environment correlation means is to point out that our *environments are heritable*. That seems like an oxymoron at first, but it definitely is not. Heritable simply means influenced by genetics. We do not experience our environments at random; they are influenced by our genotypes through gene–environment correlation. A truly remarkable recent study makes this point very strongly.[12] The focus of this study of more than 2,000 parents and their children was on educational attainment, but the concept applies equally well to psychological problems. The researchers used data from a previous study to create polygenic risk scores for educational attainment, meaning the years of education a person obtains. The fact that one can create a polygenic risk for educational attainment means that genetic variation is one of the factors that influences how many years we stay in school and the diplomas we attain. The SNPs in this polygenic risk score almost certainly influence intelligence and personality traits such as conscientiousness that are related to educational attainment. These researchers took the analysis a remarkable step further, however, and found that children who had a *higher* polygenic risk score for educational attainment than each of their parents (this can occur because each child could receive a "lucky" random draw of the polymorphic genes from each parent) showed *upward mobility* in the sense of receiving more education on average than their parents. If the polygenic risk score of the children was lower than that of their parents, however, they received less education than their parents.[12] Thus, the experience of receiving more or less education can be said to be heritable to an extent because the combined effect of the SNPs on each person was one of the influences on their educational experiences. This and other studies suggest that the experiences that shape many of our dimensions of behavior, including psychological problems, come about through gene–environment correlation.

To bring this discussion of gene–environment correlations back to the issue of psychological problems, consider two immensely important discoveries. First, a large study of adult twins found that stressful life events are influenced mostly by the same genes that influence depression.[19] Through the processes of active and evocative gene–environment correlations, those of us with a greater genetic tendency to depression tend to experience the most stress in our lives. This means that our genes are partly the unwitting architects of the stress in our lives. Perhaps this important insight can help us avoid creating our own stressors. I am not underestimating how difficult that would be for some people, but it is a possibility.

Second, if you are a parent, or may become one someday, the concept of gene–environment correlation could be of great importance to you. We usually think that the way in which we raise our children influences their behavior, and it does. But, through active and evocative gene–environmental correlations, our children's genetically influenced behavior influences our parenting as well.[20] That may be a good thing—we may sensitively respond to our children's behavior and adjust our parenting to meet their needs.[21] Nonethelesss, we have to be aware of the possibility that challenging child behavior may bring out the worst in our parenting. Unfortunately, there is considerable evidence to support this possibility.[22–24] Even the best-intentioned parents find psychological problems in their children to be challenging and do not always respond in the best ways. Having our eyes open to this possibility may help us parent better.

Gene–Environment Interactions

A different but equally important way in which genes and environments work together is through gene–environment interactions. This means that the influence of environments on our behavior depends on our genes, and conversely, the influence of our genes on our behavior depends on our environments.[18] In other words, our genetic and environmental influences to behave in a certain way do not just combine *additively*; they *multiply* the effects of one another.

Gene–Environment Interactions in Humans

Studies of adopted children have provided important information on interactions between genetic and environmental influences of psychological problems. In a study of the vast national Swedish medical registry, for example, families were identified in which at least one parent was given the diagnosis of major depression. Among those families, the investigators identified ones in which one sibling was given up for adoption and the other sibling was reared by the biological parents. Compared to the siblings raised by their own depressed biological parent(s), the adopted-away siblings had a 20% lower risk of being given the diagnosis of major depression themselves, but only when their adoptive parents never received a diagnosis of major depression and the adoptive family was not broken by divorce or parental death.[25] This suggests that the offspring's genetic risk for depression was reduced by being raised in the favorable environmental provided by well-functioning adoptive parents, but not in the less adaptive environments provided by adoptive families that did not function as well. Similar analyses by the same investigators found that the adoption of genetically high-risk children by only well-functioning families reduced risk for drug abuse and criminal behavior in the offspring.[26–28] These findings illustrate the idea that genetic predispositions interact with child-rearing environments: The degree of genetic influences on psychological problems in the adoptive children was weakened when the adoptive family functioned well and provided an adaptive child-rearing environment but not when the adoptive family did not function as well.

A recent study of genetic and environmental influences on the general factor of psychology problems also revealed a gene–environment interaction. Although most studies now examine many SNPs together, this illustrative study used a single genetic polymorphism known to be associated with psychological problems in what is termed a "candidate gene study."[29] The researchers examined a SNP in the gene that influences the receptor for the potentially important neurohormone oxytocin. Because each person inherits from each parent either an A (adenine) or a G (guanine) nucleotide at this locus in the gene, each person has an AA, AG, or GG genotype. In the Pittsburgh Girls Study, in which frequent assessments of the experiences and behavior of 2,500 girls were conducted from childhood through early adulthood, the investigators first found that stressful life events (e.g., observing community violence, witnessing domestic violence, or being the victim of physical, emotional, or sexual abuse) before age 12 years predicted higher scores on the general factor of psychological problems in early adulthood. Thus, it appears that one set of genetic and environmental factors is shared at Level 1, and two or more different sets of genetic and environmental factors are shared at Level 2. But, there was a significant gene–environment interaction: The association between more years of exposure to early stress and the adopted offspring's psychological problems was stronger for women with at least one A allele in their genotype.[29] That is, there was gene–environment interaction—the apparent effect of the environment depended on the genotype.

Another recent study of genetic and environmental influences, this time on schizophrenic behavior, also revealed a gene–environment interaction using polygenic risk scores based on many SNPs. In a sample of more than 3,000 individuals, a polygenic risk score for liability to schizophrenia and a kind of experience believed to increase risk for schizophrenia—being sexually abused during childhood—were each found to be significantly associated with the diagnosis of schizophrenia when tested individually. When the sexual abuse occurred to a person with high genetic risk for schizophrenia, however, sexual abuse was associated with the diagnosis of schizophrenia to a substantially greater extent than when sexual abuse occurred in the absence of high genetic risk.[30] Persons at high genetic risk were more influenced by the experience than were persons with lower genetic risk. Conversely, high genetic risk for schizophrenia measured by the polygenic risk score was more strongly associated with the diagnosis of schizophrenia in persons with a history of sexual abuse than in persons without this environmental risk factor.

Biological Mechanisms of Gene–Environment Interactions

Much more research is needed to fully understand gene–environment interactions in the origins of psychological problems, but a considerable amount of information from studies of nonhuman animals has both documented gene–environment interactions and revealed some important ways in which such interactions operate at the biological level of analysis. That is, these studies tell us how the outside environment can get "under the skin" and influence how genes work inside the cells of the body. There are many biological pathways through which gene–environment interactions occur,[31] including three mechanisms:

- *Environmental influences on transcription*: One biological mechanism of gene–environment interaction has been understood for many years. As discussed previously, a gene is a segment of DNA that is capable of regulating the synthesis of a protein through a number of steps beginning with gene transcription. Genes are quiescent—inactive—until something launches transcription. A substance called a transcription factor must bind with the gene for it to begin making a partial copy of the DNA sequence, called messenger RNA, which eventually determines which protein is synthesized. This is relevant, of course, because genes do not influence us unless they are transcribed and expressed. Critically, hormones released by the adrenal glands when a person is stressed regulate transcription factors. Thus, stress, which is one of the most important aspects of our experiences related to psychological problems, can influence the transcription of genes. In this way, something in our outside environment, such as a boss who is stressfully harassing us, can influence the activity of the genes inside our cells. It is important to note, however, that not everyone's genes are equally likely to be transcribed. Because some forms of polymorphic genes are more easily transcribed than others,[32] our genetic variation can even influence the impact of transcription factors on genes. This provides another mechanism of gene–environment interaction.
- *Epigenetic modification of the genome*: Scientists have recently learned that the experiences of nonhuman mammals can make their genes more or less susceptible to transcription factors. Our experiences can lead some complex molecules to bind to our DNA sequences, changing how likely they are to be expressed and begin the process of protein synthesis in the presence of transcription factors. For example, when methyl molecules bind to certain C (cytosine) nucleotides in the DNA sequence, they "silence" the gene by making it less open to transcription.

In contrast, the binding of acetyl molecules to other parts of the strand of DNA makes the gene more open to translation. Such modification of the likelihood of gene expression provides another pathway for gene–environment interaction. Environmental events, such as stress or atypical maternal care, can influence DNA methylation, muting or silencing some genes. Thus, genes and environments can interact because our experiences can influence how much our genetic variants can influence us.[33] This process is even more nuanced in the sense that some variants of polymorphic genes are more subject to methylation that others.[34] The key issue here is that our external environments and variations in our DNA sequences influence our behavior interactively through methylation and other modifications of the openness of genes to transcription.

These findings are enormously important, but the full story of gene–environment interaction at the biological level is even more amazing. In studies of rat pups, the methylation of some genes was found to be influenced by the ways in which they were cared for by their mothers. In turn, these methylated genes influenced how responsive the rat pups were to stress when they matured. You may want to sit down now because the next part is just astonishing. Michael Meaney and colleagues[35] found that some of the DNA methylation caused by variations in maternal care can be passed down to the *next generation* and influence their stress responsiveness! This means that a characteristic acquired in one generation—methylation of a gene that reduces responsiveness to stress—was "inherited" by the next generation. The word inherited is in quotes in the previous sentence because it is not based on variations in the DNA sequence, which is the classical basis for inheritance.[36]

This nongenetic kind of inheritance was believed to be impossible until only recently. Most of us accept the theory of inheritance through natural selection that evolved from the work of Charles Darwin and Gregor Mendel, which eventually spawned the discovery of the role of DNA in inheritance by Franklin, Crick, and Watson.[37] Modern Darwinian theory states that some mutations in the DNA sequence that help organisms survive and successfully reproduce are preferentially passed on to the next generation, forming the genetic basis of evolution. In contrast, Jean Baptiste Lamarck published a theory of evolution in 1801, 58 years before Darwin's *On the Origin of Species*. He posited that characteristics acquired in one generation are passed to the next generation; for example, longer necks thought to be caused by stretching for food in trees by giraffes are passed to the next generation, resulting in progressively longer necks in giraffes. Lamarck's theory was largely ignored after Darwin's theory was published, but several writers have suggested that he has risen from the grave to give congratulatory slaps on the back of Michael Meaney!

Lest we be too quick to accept the idea that inherited methylation that influences gene expression is related to psychological problems, we need to remember that although the finding in rats has been replicated in other nonhuman animals,[37] we do not yet know if it applies to humans. Moreover, no one is giving up on classic views of the role of DNA in inheritance just yet. These studies showed that experiences in one generation can change the methylation of DNA, but they do not change the DNA sequence. Or do they? Yes, well, if you like scientific revolutions, read on:

- *Genetic retrotransposition*: The third way that environmental experiences can interact with DNA involves actual *changes in the DNA sequence* caused by experiences. You read that correctly! About one-third of our DNA is composed of segments that are mobile. The mobile DNA segments that seem to be most important in humans are called *retrotransposons*. Recently, it has been found that low levels of adaptive maternal care can cause movement of retrotransposons to new positions in the DNA in the brains of rats, changing the DNA sequence.[38] Relatively little is known about the role of retrotransposition in gene–environment interaction in humans, but changes in the positions of retrotransposons are known to alter gene expression in nonhuman animals.[39] Notably, such changes in DNA sequence may be passed to the next generation if they occur in sperm or egg cells.[40] These experience-caused changes in DNA sequence do not throw our understanding of genetics out the window, but they certainly make it a more complex and interesting topic.

Darwin is safe for now, but brushing up on Larmarck might be a good idea.

To avoid missing the forest for the trees here, let me remind you that the take-home message is that genes and environments work together, through both gene–environment correlations and gene–environment interactions. We never have to ask if risk for a kind of psychological problem is influenced by genes or environments; the answer is always that both work together. With that in mind, let us return to the concept of heritability to reveal more about the environmental side of the interplay of genes and environments.

Heritability and Two Kinds of Environments

When twin researchers were developing the concept of heritability (i.e., the proportion of variation in any phenotype due to genetic influences), they also very insightfully distinguished between two kinds of environments.[41] This distinction has proven to be extremely useful in a number of ways when we think about human welfare, so it deserves careful consideration. I hinted at this distinction in Chapter 6, but I elaborate on it here to help us understand the concept of heritability. *Shared environments* are the same for all siblings in a family. If siblings are raised by the same biological parents in the same home and the same neighborhood, those are aspects of their environments that the siblings share. Factors related to race, poverty, and neighborhoods are generally shared environments. In contrast, *nonshared environments* are the things that happen to one sibling but not the other or are different for the siblings. For example, if one sibling is physically assaulted and the other is not, that constitutes an unshared environmental influence on one sibling. Shared environments can make siblings more similar, but nonshared environments understandably can make them different.

When I say that the heritability of a phenotype such as the diagnosis of schizophrenia behavior is estimated to be 80%, that sounds like there is little room for the environment to play a role. I have already told you that is not true, but I need to tell you more about heritability estimates to explain why. Some kinds of gene–environment interactions increase the estimate of heritability. If something in the shared environment has a powerful effect but does so by interacting with polymorphic genes, that effect adds to the estimate of heritability. For example, to use a hypothetical example, if cold parenting were shared equally by all siblings in a family but increased risk for later depression only in siblings with a particular high-risk genotype, that would constitute a gene–environment interaction. Nonetheless, it would count toward the estimate of heritability. That is because all of the siblings experience the same parenting in this example, and only the genetic effect (i.e., the difference between the siblings in genotype) is observed. Because such gene–environment interactions are likely to be important, our shared experiences may well play a more important role than implied by the high heritability estimates for most dimension of psychological problems.

Environments that Contribute to Psychological Problems

It has been remarkably difficult for psychologists to discover the specific environments that cause psychological problems. Gene–environment correlations mean that environments are confounded with genes to such a degree that it is very difficult to tease them apart. If you compare three large groups of people who became artists, farmers, or accountants as adults and find that the artists were much more likely to take art classes in high school, you could not conclude that high school art classes led them into a career in art. Why not? That might seem like a reasonable explanation, but we would need to know more. The artists could differ genetically from the farmers and accountants, and those genes might have both influenced their career choice and, through selective gene–environment correlation, led them to take high school art classes. Thus, any apparent effect of taking art classes on career choice could be the result of the same genotype influencing both taking art classes and career choices. For this reason, it is difficult to rule out genetic confounds when trying to identify environments that increase risk for psychological problems. This topic is discussed further in Chapter 9.

References

1. Sandin S, Lichtenstein P, Kuja-Halkola R, Hultman C, Larsson H, Reichenberg A. The heritability of autism spectrum disorder. *JAMA.* 2017;318(12):1182–1184.

2. Hilker R, Helenius D, Fagerlund B, et al. Heritability of schizophrenia and schizophrenia spectrum based on the nationwide Danish Twin Register. *Biological Psychiatry.* 2018;83(6):492–498.

3. Merwood A, Greven CU, Price TS, et al. Different heritabilities but shared etiological influences for parent, teacher and self-ratings of ADHD symptoms: An adolescent twin study. *Psychological Medicine.* 2013;43(9):1973–1984.

4. Larsson H, Chang Z, D'Onofrio BM, Lichtenstein P. The heritability of clinically diagnosed attention deficit hyperactivity disorder across the lifespan. *Psychological Medicine.* 2014;44(10):2223–2229.

5. Heath AC, Bucholz KK, Madden PAF, et al. Genetic and environmental contributions to alcohol dependence risk in a national twin sample: Consistency of findings in women and men. *Psychological Medicine.* 1997;27(6):1381–1396.

6. Hettema JM, Neale MC, Kendler KS. A review and meta-analysis of the genetic epidemiology of anxiety disorders. *American Journal of Psychiatry.* 2001;158(10):1568–1578.

7. Bierut LJ, Heath AC, Bucholz KK, et al. Major depressive disorder in a community-based twin sample—Are there different genetic and environmental contributions for men and women? *Archives of General Psychiatry.* 1999;56(6):557–563.

8. Kendler KS, Gardner CO, Neale MC, Prescott CA. Genetic risk factors for major depression in men and women: Similar or different heritabilities and same or partly distinct genes? *Psychological Medicine.* 2001;31(4):605–616.

9. Cardno AG, Gottesman, II. Twin studies of schizophrenia: From bow-and-arrow concordances to Star Wars Mx and functional genomics. *American Journal of Medical Genetics.* 2000;97(1):12–17.

10. Janssens ACJW. Validity of polygenic risk scores: Are we measuring what we think we are? *Human Molecular Genetics.* 2019;28(R2):R143–R150.

11. Agerbo E, Sullivan PF, Vilhjalmsson BJ, et al. Polygenic risk score, parental socioeconomic status, family history of psychiatric disorders, and the risk for schizophrenia: A Danish population-based study and meta-analysis. *JAMA Psychiatry.* 2015;72(7):635–641.

12. McGue M, Willoughby EA, Rustichini A, Johnson W, Iacono WG, Lee JJ. The contribution of cognitive and noncognitive skills to intergenerational social mobility *Psychological Science*. 2020;31(7):835–847.

13. Lahey BB, Van Hulle CA, Singh AL, Waldman ID, Rathouz PJ. Higher-order genetic and environmental structure of prevalent forms of child and adolescent psychopathology. *Archives of General Psychiatry*. 2011;68:181–189.

14. Lahey BB, Krueger RF, Rathouz PJ, Waldman ID, Zald DH. A hierarchical causal taxonomy of psychopathology across the life span. *Psychological Bulletin*. 2017;143:142–186.

15. Lee R, Garcia F, van de Kar LD, Hauger RD, Coccaro EF. Plasma oxytocin in response to pharmaco-challenge to D-fenfluramine and placebo in healthy men. *Psychiatry Research*. 2003;118:129–136.

16. Riglin L, Thapar AK, Leppert B, et al. Using genetics to examine a general liability to childhood psychopathology. *Behavior Genetics*. 2020;50(4):213–220.

17. Smoller JW, Andreassen OA, Edenberg HJ, Faraone SV, Glatt SJ, Kendler KS. Psychiatric genetics and the structure of psychopathology. *Molecular Psychiatry*. 2019;24(3):409–420.

18. Plomin R, DeFries JC, Loehlin JC. Genotype–environment interaction and correlation in the analysis of human behavior. *Psychological Bulletin*. 1977;84:309–322.

19. Kendler KS, Gardner CO. Depressive vulnerability, stressful life events and episode onset of major depression: A longitudinal model. *Psychological Medicine*. 2016;46(9):1865–1874.

20. Ayoub M, Briley DA, Grotzinger A, et al. Genetic and environmental associations between child personality and parenting. *Social Psychological and Personality Science*. 2019;10(6):711–721.

21. Cheung AK, Harden KP, Tucker-Drob EM. Multivariate behavioral genetic analysis of parenting in early childhood. *Parenting-Science and Practice*. 2016;16(4):257–283.

22. Abel KM, Drake R, Goldstein JM. Sex differences in schizophrenia. *International Review of Psychiatry*. 2010;22(5):417–428.

23. Flom M, White D, Ganiban J, Saudino KJ. Longitudinal links between callous-unemotional behaviors and parenting in early childhood: A genetically informed design. *Journal of the American Academy of Child and Adolescent Psychiatry*. 2020;59(3):401–409.e2.

24. Bilsky SA, Cole DA, Dukewich TL, et al. Does supportive parenting mitigate the longitudinal effects of peer victimization on depressive thoughts and symptoms in children? *Journal of Abnormal Psychology*. 2013;122(2):406–419.

25. Kendler KS, Ohlsson H, Sundquist J, Sundquist K. The rearing environment and risk for major depression: A Swedish national high-risk

home-reared and adopted-away co-sibling control study. *American Journal of Psychiatry.* 2020;177(5):447–453.

26. Kendler KS, Morris NA, Ohlsson H, Lonn SL, Sundquist J, Sundquist K. Criminal offending and the family environment: Swedish national high-risk home-reared and adopted-away co-sibling control study. *British Journal of Psychiatry.* 2016;209(4):296–301.

27. Kendler KS, Ohlsson H, Sundquist K, Sundquist J. The rearing environment and risk for drug abuse: A Swedish national high-risk adopted and not adopted co-sibling control study. *Psychological Medicine.* 2016;46(7):1359–1366.

28. Kendler KS, Turkheimer E, Ohlsson H, Sundquist J, Sundquist K. Family environment and the malleability of cognitive ability: A Swedish national home-reared and adopted-away cosibling control study. *Proceedings of the National Academy of Sciences of the United States of America.* 2015;112(15):4612–4617.

29. Byrd AL, Tung I, Manuck SB, et al. An interaction between early threat exposure and the oxytocin receptor in females: Disorder-specific versus general risk for psychopathology and social–emotional mediators. *Development and Psychopathology.* 2020:1–16.

30. Guloksuz S, Pries LK, Delespaul P, et al. Examining the independent and joint effects of molecular genetic liability and environmental exposures in schizophrenia: Results from the EUGEI study. *World Psychiatry.* 2019;18(2):173–182.

31. Roberts BW, Jackson JJ. Sociogenomic personality psychology. *Journal of Personality.* 2008;76(6):1523–1544.

32. Donaldson ZR, le Francois B, Santos TL, et al. The functional serotonin 1a receptor promoter polymorphism, rs6295, is associated with psychiatric illness and differences in transcription. *Translational Psychiatry.* 2016;6:e746.

33. Turecki G, Meaney MJ. Effects of the social environment and stress on glucocorticoid receptor gene methylation: A systematic review. *Biological Psychiatry.* 2016;79(2):87–96.

34. Czamara D, Eraslan G, Page CM, et al. Integrated analysis of environmental and genetic influences on cord blood DNA methylation in newborns. *Nature Communications.* 2019;10:548.

35. Meaney, M. J. Maternal care, gene expression, and the transmission of individual differences in stress reactivity across generations. *Annual Review of Neuroscience.* 2001;24:1161–1192.

36. Watson JD, Crick FHC. A structure for deoxyribose nucleic acid. *Nature.* 1953;171:737–738

37. Franklin TB, Russig H, Weiss IC, et al. Epigenetic transmission of the impact of early stress across generations. *Biological Psychiatry.* 2010;68(5):408–415.

38. Bedrosian TA, Quayle C, Novaresi N, Gage FH. Early life experience drives structural variation of neural genomes in mice. *Science.* 2018;359(6382):1395–1399.
39. Elbarbary RA, Lucas BA, Maquat LE. Retrotransposons as regulators of gene expression. *Science.* 2016;351(6274):aac7247.
40. Chuong EB, Elde NC, Feschotte C. Regulatory activities of transposable elements: From conflicts to benefits. *Nature Reviews Genetics.* 2017;18(2):71–86.
41. Rowe DC, Plomin R. The importance of non-shared (E1) environmental influences in behavioral development. *Developmental Psychology.* 1981;17(5):517–531.

9

Ordinary Origins of
Psychological Problems

Transacting with the World

In Chapter 8, I summarized some of what has been learned about the natural and ubiquitous interplay of genetic and environmental influences on psychological problems. This chapter goes deeper into the role of environmental influences, but without forgetting that environmental influences always play their role in the context of gene–environment correlations and interactions. With that in mind, it is almost certainly correct to say that the ways in which we act, think, and feel—whether they are adaptive or problematic—are influenced in perfectly ordinary ways by experiences in our environments. That is a more controversial, complex, and interesting statement than it may first appear, however.

Environments

To understand how our environments influence our risk for psychological problems, I first summarize research on the specific kinds of experiences that research tells us put people at high risk for psychological problems. Then I present some potentially important hypotheses regarding the specific processes through which our environments give rise to psychological problems.

High-Risk Environments

It is essential to keep two things in mind as we discuss high-risk environments. First, although it is relatively easy to determine if some aspect of the environment is statistically associated with psychological problems, it is much more difficult to conclude that the environment *causes* psychological problems. This is partly because high-risk environments are complex, with many different environmental risk factors co-occurring that are difficult to tease apart. Furthermore, the genetic characteristics of persons who live in high-risk environments tend to differ from those who live in low-risk environments. Genes and environments are correlated, making it difficult to isolate the role of particular parts of the environment. Furthermore, environments likely influence different people in different ways due to gene–environment interactions.

Another way of saying this is that high-risk environments are always *confounded* by many other factors. It is relatively easy to distinguish among confounded risk factors by conducting true experiments, but we cannot ethically conduct such studies of environmental risk factors for psychological problems. A true experiment would require us to randomly assign some people to live in a high-risk environment and others to live in benign environments. For example, for obvious reasons, we would not randomly assign some children to have terrible experiences such as the death of a parent to see if they develop psychological problems. Therefore, we have to make clever use of the data that we can collect ethically and carefully and tentatively draw the best conclusions we can.

Keep in mind that we are talking about average statistical associations between environments and psychological problems. Not everyone who lives in high-risk environments has psychological problems, whereas many people from low-risk environments do have problems. With those caveats in mind, here is a summary of what is currently known about the high-risk environments that are associated with psychological problems.

Stressful Experiences

Life is great, isn't it? Well, it often is great, but not all the time. Challenges and misfortunes are almost inevitable, with some of us being exposed to far more stress than others. Persons who experience acutely stressful events, such as being raped, assaulted, bullied, fired from a job, being wounded in combat, or losing a loved one, are more likely to experience psychological problems.[1-6] In a long-term study of some 2,000 adolescents in the Netherlands,[7] for example, four times as many youth who experienced the death of a family member subsequently experienced an increase in depression and anxiety than youth who were not bereaved. And there is clear evidence that persons who are abused or victimized—physically or sexually—are more likely to experience a broad range of psychological problems in childhood and adulthood.[8-10] Even people who just experience prolonged mild stressors and hassles are more likely to develop depression and other psychological problems.[11-13]

There was a dramatic rise in serious stressors during the time in which this book was written during 2020 and early 2021. People all over the world confronted the multiple stressors involved in the novel COVID-19 pandemic. Many people were stressed by the threat of illness and death, the loss of loved ones, the loss of income, the disruption of routines and social support, and by witnessing the terrible inequities in the impact of COVID-19 on people of color. The pandemic resulted in increases in anxiety, depression, and thinking about suicide in many persons.[14,15] At the same time, we witnessed the unspeakably wrong killings of Black Americans by police during the same year. In addition, many people in the United States have begun to experience the stressors that have arisen from global warming, particularly from unprecedented heat and drought turning forests into tinder that burns disastrously. People in low-lying coastal regions and islands in the United States and many other countries have already been sorely stressed by rising waters. Tragically, the stressors from global warming will be orders of magnitude worse than even the COVID-19 pandemic for many people. Unless we take drastic actions to protect the environment now, billions of people will be stressed when rising waters reach their doors and soaring temperatures dry out croplands, causing mass starvation and armed conflicts over food in many areas of the world. Recent events are making an increasing number of people realize that human beings are an endangered species.

Discrimination

It is very important to call attention to a kind of stress than the majority of people do not, by definition, experience because most of us are in the majority. People who have a different color of skin, are from a different culture, or who practice different religions than most people in their communities often experience stressful discrimination. The same is true for those who are sexually attracted to their own sex or who define their gender and dress in ways that are out of the gendered mainstream. Being different anywhere on earth can subject you to abuse. People who are in the minority in some way know this very well, but most people who are in the majority have not given the stressful experiences of discrimination enough credence. It is difficult to put oneself in the shoes of others, of course, and it is understandable that majority scientists have studied the kinds of stressors that they experience themselves. Yet, our slowness to study the stressfulness of discrimination smacks of unconscious, or even willful, neglect by those of us who enjoy the privileges of the majority. It is uncomfortable to learn that our behavior hurts other people through both our own direct actions and the discriminatory practices of police, courts, banks, and elected officials that we tacitly support with our silence. Fortunately, psychologists have recently conducted studies that demonstrate that the experience of being discriminated against is stressful.[16] Although this should come as no surprise to anyone, such studies may make the stress of discrimination more difficult to ignore.

Economic Hardship

The members of families living in conditions of economic hardship are more likely to experience psychological problems than members of more affluent families.[17–19] By itself, this association does not tell us that a life constrained by inadequate economic resources causes psychological problems, of course. For one thing, the direction of causation could be in the opposite direction. We know that people with serious psychological problems terminate their education early and have lower incomes as adults than people with fewer problems,[20] so it is possible that psychological problems cause lower family income rather than—or in addition to—the opposite. Nonetheless, there is increasingly strong evidence that economic hardships do *cause* psychological problems. The worldwide Great Recession that occurred in 2008 because of the collapse of unwise and illegal mortgage lending brought about dramatic increases in unemployment, personal debt, bankruptcy, and housing evictions and foreclosures. The well-documented fact that depression, anxiety, and suicide increased soon after economic hardships increased during this economic recession strongly supports the hypothesis that declines in economic resources cause psychological problems.[21–23]

Furthermore, several researchers have used clever statistical analyses to strengthen the conclusion that living in a family with few economic resources *causes* an increase in psychological problems, particularly when they experience poverty as children.[24] One study used a large sample of mothers who were representative of young women in the United States.[25] The families were interviewed multiple times as the children grew through adolescence. Controlling for birth order and other factors, the investigators compared the psychological problems of the children in the family who were exposed to lower family incomes when they were young to their siblings who were young during times of higher family income. Children in families who were exposed to poverty when they were young had more conduct problems than their more fortunate siblings. This suggests that something about being a young child in an impoverished family causes conduct problems. Comparing siblings within the same families rules out many, but not all, potential confounds and alternative explanations. Studies like these substantially strengthen the case that early poverty is psychologically toxic to young children.

Another study used a very different strategy to draw causal inferences about changes in family income. Children living on a Native American reservation were studied before and after their families began receiving cash payments from the tribe due to the opening of a tribal casino.[26] When family incomes increased because of these payments, conduct problems in the children decreased. Because the change in income was completely unrelated to the genetic and other characteristics of the families, this provides evidence that increasing family incomes caused an improvement in behavior problems in their children. Other studies have found that simple cash transfers from the federal government to low-income citizens during times of economic hardship, similar to the cash transfers given in the United States during the coronavirus pandemic, reduce intimate partner violence and suicide.[24] Every citizen should know that very easily administered anti-poverty programs such as cash transfers can reduce poverty and thereby reduce psychological problems and their downstream consequences (missed work, greater medical costs, etc.) on society. In wealthy countries, having part of the population live in poverty is a choice of the society; it is not an inevitability. And it is a very costly choice to everyone in society in the long term.

How could low family income cause psychological problems in children? Parents under economic pressure cannot pay for adequate food and other basic needs, fall behind in payments and face growing debt, worry about losing their homes to foreclosure, and may experience periods of homelessness. One influential theory posits that these events lead to unhappy and irritable parents who tend to interact joylessly and coercively with their children.[27] In addition, the children may experience reductions in adult supervision if parents have to work multiple low-paying jobs to make ends meet, and they may be embarrassed by their old clothes and the like. These factors combine to increase the risk for conduct problems in the children.

Disorganized Neighborhoods

Psychological problems, such as antisocial behavior, drug use, and depression, are more common among the residents of disorganized and unsafe neighborhoods.[28,29] Disorganized neighborhoods are ones in which the residents do not work together effectively to solve problems, from the lack of streetlights to violence and open drug selling. There is growing evidence that our psychological problems are influenced by characteristics of the neighborhoods we live in.[30] For example, exposure to violence in a distressed neighborhood may directly promote anxiety and depression,[31] and living in neighborhoods with higher concentrations of antisocial and drug-using youth creates more opportunities to socialize adolescents into drug use and delinquency.[32,33]

An unusual and highly informative true experiment called Moving to Opportunity was conducted by the U.S. Department of Housing and Urban Development to evaluate the benefits of moving families from distressed to less distressed neighborhoods. Some residents of disorganized low-income neighborhoods were selected by random lottery to receive government financial assistance to allow them to move to less distressed neighborhoods. During the next 10–15 years, the physical and mental health of the families who moved were compared to those of families not randomly selected to move to better neighborhoods. The change to a more advantaged neighborhood was associated with fewer psychological problems, better health, and a greater subjective sense of well-being in the family members.[34]

Polluted and Diminished Physical Environments

There is increasing evidence that the physical environments that we create are associated with the likelihood of psychological problems. Living in an area of high air pollution, particularly high levels of nitrogen dioxide and small particulate matter, is associated with higher rates of depression, bipolar disorder, and psychotic experiences.[35,36] Conversely, greater neighborhood greenness—the presence of grass, bushes, and trees—is associated with less depression in the residents.[28] These are very compelling findings, but it is not yet clear if these aspects of the physical environment actually influence the likelihood of psychological problems. Fortunately, there are plenty of good health and environmental reasons to reduce air pollution everywhere, and it never hurts to plant trees and bushes.

Environmental Influences on Psychological Problems

How do we acquire psychological problems from our environments? Much remains to be learned, but it is very likely that our environments affect us in two ways:

1. *Reactions to stress*: Sometimes our emotional reactions to the pummeling of stress directly amount to psychological problems. Stress can directly make us tense, worried, sad, disinterested, and keep us up at night. When enduring, those and other reactions to stress may be upsetting enough or interfere with our daily activities enough to warrant considering them to be psychological problems.

2. *Learning*: The second way in which our environments can cause psychological problems is through learning. Throughout our lives, we learn from our experiences. Sometimes what we learn is adaptive, but sometimes we learn maladaptive behavior—ways of acting, thinking, feeling, and believing that cause us grief; psychological problems, in other words.

We learn from our environments in three major ways. First, we learn by *observing* others in our environments; new ways of behaving spread through communities largely because one person imitates another, usually without thinking about it. Psychological problems linked to the use of new street drugs, for example, may spread in this way. Seeing someone enjoy a drug may lead others to try it.

Second, we learn from the *consequences* of our behavior. When we behave in a way that leads to a positive consequence, that usually makes us more likely to act that way again in the future. For example, if a person complains loudly and dramatically about minor aches and pains and gets an unusual amount of help and sympathy from people who usually ignore them, that positive outcome may increase the likelihood of somatic complaints in the future. Similarly, a child walking to school who is frightened by a tethered dog that barks aggressively may feel a reduction in fear when they take a longer route to school the next day. Unfortunately, the positive consequence of experiencing less fear may not only make the child more likely to take the long way to school but also strengthen the fear of dogs.

Third, we sometimes acquire maladaptive behavior through *association*. Through this simple form of learning, some part of our world may come to elicit a positive or negative emotional reaction that it is not actually related to that reaction. For example, a person who walks past a mountain laurel bush in the woods and sees a frightening rattlesnake may react with irrational fear to mountain laurels in the future, even in settings in which snakes are scarce.

These three kinds of learning can affect us profoundly, even when we do not consciously notice the learning process taking place.[37,38]

Transactions

Everything I have just said about experiences that foster psychological problems is correct, but it is an oversimplification. It is more complete and accurate to posit that psychological problems are learned as we *transact* with the environment.[39] As you read this section on transactions, keep in mind what you learned in the previous chapter about gene–environment correlations and gene–environment interactions. Those concepts are first cousins to the concept of transactions and differ only by considering the role of genetics more explicitly. This section on transactions should both flesh out our discussion of how we learn from our environments and bolster our understanding of gene–environment correlations and gene–environment interactions.

The concept of *transactions* between our behavior and our environments evolved from a seminal paper written more than 50 years ago by Robert Bell.[13] Bell was studying the interactions of parents and their young children at a time when psychologists in the Western world fervently believed that human behavior, both adaptive and maladaptive, was solely shaped by our environments, particularly the socializing experiences provided by our parents. Socialization was thought to be a one-way street in the 1960s. Bell observed, however, that parents adjusted how they interacted with their children as they responded to their children's behavior. When their children were all happy smiles, moms were far more positive with them than when their children were fussy and irritable. As a result, Bell courageously went against the prevailing wisdom in psychology and hypothesized that children influence their parents as much as parents influence their children. Gradually, his ideas took hold and were advocated by others. Although they used different terminology, Gerald Patterson[40] and Arnold Sameroff[41] elaborated Bell's idea to hypothesize that socialization is a

two-way street—children learn from their parents, but they reciprocally influence their parents' behavior toward them.

A particularly clever experiment reveals just how much parental
behavior is influenced by their child's behavior. In psychologist Hugh
Lytton's laboratory at the University of Calgary,[42] two groups of
mothers of same-age elementary school boys were observed during
three 15-minute sessions while they interacted with their own child
in one session and with another mother's child in each of the other
two sessions. Half of the children in this study had been referred to
a mental health clinic because of their serious conduct problems and
half were well-behaved children. In each session, the boys were allowed
to play freely for 5 minutes, then asked by the mothers to clean up the
toys and complete arithmetic problems. The clever part of this study
was that after they interacted with their own child, the mothers were
observed with someone else's child—for 15 minutes with a child who
exhibited conduct problems and for 15 minutes with a well-behaved
child. The mothers did not know which of the other children had been
referred to a mental health clinic for conduct problems, but when the
mothers were observed with the well-behaved children they issued
fewer commands and were less critical than when they were with a
badly behaved child. That is, the mothers of well-behaved boys started
behaving like the mothers of badly behaved children, displaying the
coercive and negative behaviors that were once thought to be the sole
cause of conduct problems in children. Parenting practices are important to be sure, but to a considerable extent, they are caused by the behavior of the child. It is a two-way street.

Thus, just as the world acts on us, we act on the world. We are not
passive blank tablets on which our psychological experiences write.
Rather, we are active determinants of our experiences. We literally
change our own worlds, and we do so on a daily if not a moment-to-
moment basis. People who interact with neighbors in a friendly and responsible way are more likely to live in a friendly neighborhood that is
partly of their own creation. People who are irresponsible, unfriendly,
and complain about unimportant things to everyone in earshot often
create unfriendly neighbors. We influence our experiences to a considerable and important extent, but it is very important to acknowledge
that there are limits on how much we can create our own environments.

Children can profoundly influence how adults and peers react to them—influencing their experiences with those people—but they have little influence on whether their parents are rich or poor, decide to divorce, use crack, or die from opioid overdose. Even adults are limited in how much they can adaptively influence their worlds by the constraints imposed on them by racism and poverty. It is not always possible to move out of high-crime neighborhoods, for example. Safe neighborhoods are expensive and guarded by insidious and invisible racist barriers in many cases. Nonetheless, within such constraints, we play an active role in creating the worlds that influence us.

Personal Characteristics and Transactions

To restate my point in other words for emphasis, we are all engaged in a dance with our environments. The world influences our next step, and we (partly) influence the next moves taken by our worlds. That is, we are constantly *transacting* with our environments and sometimes developing psychological problems in the process. What is *our* role in these transactions with the environment? Which of our personal characteristics influence our environments? In considering these questions, it is very important to note that the personal characteristics that influence our environments often also influence *how our experiences influence us*. Not everyone responds to stressors and learning experiences in the same way, and the things about us that influence our experiences are often the same things that moderate or exaggerate our responses to our experiences.

We first need to acknowledge an unsettling reality: Our sex and gender, age, skin color, physical attractiveness, style of dress, immigration status, and language influence how neighbors, teachers, store clerks, and police officers interact with us. Similarly, people of different ages experience different worlds. The interactions of children are often with adults, and even their interactions with other children are typically under adult supervision. These restrictions dictate the kinds of transactions that they experience with the world. As children age, interactions with peers become more common, and transactions with parents, day care workers, and teachers become less common. Adults interact with still different aspects of the world, including employers and their own children. Sex differences in experiences and in reactions to experiences were described in Chapter 8. Much remains to be learned about the important role of all such demographic factors in the origins of psychological problems, however.

Dispositions and Transactions

Our typical ways of behaving, often referred to as *dispositions*, also play a key role in the transactional process. I use the term disposition to mean essentially the same thing as a personality or temperament trait, but without the theoretical baggage that often accompanies those terms.[43] Throughout our lives, we learn from our teachers, peers, fellow employees, and bosses, and we reciprocally influence their behavior toward us. Crucially, our dispositional traits both shape the world in which we live and influence how we react to our experiences.

Not surprisingly, psychologists have devoted a great deal of time trying to find the best way to describe and define the dispositions that transact with our environments and make us who we are. This focus on dispositions is nothing new—Hippocrates studied personality traits around 400 BCE and Ivan Pavlov, who is best known for his work on classical conditioning, also studied dispositional traits in the late 1800s to understand why the dogs in his studies varied so much in their learning and in their behavior in and out of the laboratory.

Today, a great many psychologists still spend the better part of their working days studying this topic. It is surprising, therefore, that no consensus has been reached among psychologists about how to describe the basic human dispositional traits. There are two reasons for this. First, if I may wax metaphorical to make a point, Mother Nature assiduously guards her secrets about the workings of human nature. The nature of the traits that dispose us to acquire psychological problems through our transactions with our worlds is just one of the important things that we have not completely figured out yet. Second, the goal of science is to progressively improve the accuracy of our understanding of nature by carefully examining the findings and conclusions of others and, often as not, disagreeing with one another. This sometimes uncomfortable process of disagreement among scientists pushes us to more accurate understandings of what we study. We are still not in agreement about the most important dispositions, but we are learning more and more.

The lack of consensus among psychologists on the specific number and nature of the dispositional traits that should be distinguished to best understand humans poses a dilemma for me as I write this book. I could adopt one of the more popular models of dispositional traits, but whatever list of dispositions I adopted would please some experts and upset others. Therefore, I will not make any pronouncements about which model of dispositional traits is the best. Rather, I use some examples of dispositional traits that seem particularly important to me to make some general points about dispositions. If, and when, the field agrees on one list of human dispositions, I feel certain that the general points I make in this chapter will still apply. The important message here is that our dispositional traits make us more or less likely to develop psychological problems, largely through transactional processes. The disagreements among psychologists on the number and nature of those dispositional traits are much less important than this general idea.

Two additional points should be made about dispositions. First, although most psychologists and psychiatrists make a distinction between dispositions and psychological problems, both terms actually refer to the same thing—our behavior. Nonetheless, I personally think that distinguishing between dispositional traits and dimensions of psychological problems can help us understand the transactional process. Second, I think we can confidently hypothesize a strong and revealing link between dispositions and the important topics of gene–environment correlation and interaction discussed in Chapter 8. Each of the dispositional traits described in this section is moderately heritable, meaning that they are influenced by polymorphic genes.[44] It seems very likely to me that the genetically influenced characteristics of persons that drive active and evocative gene–environment correlations and play a role in gene–environment interactions involve these dispositional traits. With these two points in mind, let us consider some of the dispositional traits that seem to play important roles in our learning adaptive or maladaptive behavior through transactions with the environment.[45]

Negative Emotionality versus Emotional Stability

It makes sense to begin our discussion with a dispositional trait that is recognized by essentially every theorist. Negative emotionality, which is often referred to using the older term of neuroticism, refers to individual differences in how we respond with negative emotions to stressors—to our losses, frustrations, hassles, pressures, and threats. Everyone experiences stress, but we react to it in different ways. Some people remain placid in the face of stress; but people who are high on the disposition of negative emotionality have low thresholds for stress, respond frequently and intensely to stress with negative emotions, and recover more slowly after the stress ends. These negative emotions include everything from fear to depression to anger, with the particular negative emotions evoked depending on the nature of the stressor, the circumstances, and other characteristics of the individual. In some individuals who are high in dispositional negative emotionality, stress elicits some combination of worry, muscle tension, irritability, sadness, loss of pleasure and enjoyment, and disruption of key housekeeping functions of the body—sleeping and eating. Other individuals high in negative emotionality respond to stress with tantrums, anger, stubbornness, and uncontrolled aggression. The key thing is that people high in negative emotionality have a low threshold for stressful events, respond intensely to them in some way, and return to a calm state slowly.[46,47]

Most important for our purposes, people who are high on the disposition of negative emotionality are at increased risk for psychological problems. An analysis of studies involving repeated psychological assessments of more than 400,000 people over many years has shown that persons who are higher in negative emotionality are considerably more likely to develop a wide variety of new psychological problems over the next few years.[48]

Why does the extent to which each person responds to aversive events with negative emotions predict their likelihood of developing psychological problems? Persons who are higher in negative emotionality have a bias for paying attention to negative information—they notice more of the bad things in life, giving themselves more opportunities to respond with negative emotions,[46] and are particularly sensitive to signs of rejection by others.[49,50] Furthermore, negative emotionality influences how easily we *learn* psychological problems from our transactions with the world in two ways. First, negative emotions sometimes provide the "raw material" that our experiences shape into psychological problems. Imagine a scenario involving a child who is high in negative emotionality: The child responds to a request to pick up their toys with a loud "No!" and stamped feet. The child's father counters with a firm, "Oh, yes, you will," which elicits additional negative emotional responses from the child, such as a raging temper tantrum, complete with hitting the father and throwing toys. Imagine that the father turns his back and walks away from this aversive exchange, saying "Have it your way! I don't care if your room is a mess." What is the likely effect of this transaction on the child? The child has been reinforced for responding with intense emotions and is likely learning the psychological problem of oppositional behavior to the reasonable requests of adults. The child's dispositional negative emotions were the behavioral raw material from which specific oppositional and aggressive behaviors were shaped through transactions with a parent.

Furthermore, this child probably influenced their future parenting environment through this transaction—the father may be less likely to make appropriate requests in the future. This means that the child will have fewer opportunities to learn to be cooperative with parents. When adults try to play a constructive role in the lives of children who are high in negative emotionality, they often find themselves involved in coercive exchanges with the child that can result in their backing down from their reasonable requests, giving in, and reinforcing child noncompliance at home and school.[51] Similarly, negative emotional responses to provocations (e.g., when another child plays with a toy that the emotional child wants) can lead other children to defer, reinforcing their antisocial behavior. The net result is that negative emotionality promotes the learning of maladaptive behaviors.

That is only one example of how being characteristically high in negative emotionality increases the risk of developing psychological problems, however. For example, negative emotionality also influences how easily we learn irrational fears through the process of association.[46] That single hypothetical encounter with a mountain laurel bush and a snake that I described previously would not classically condition everyone to have a phobia of bushes, but persons high in negative emotionality develop conditioned fears particularly easily.[46]

Prosociality versus Callousness

Prosociality refers to a disposition to care about the welfare of others, attempt to help and please them, and experience guilt over misbehaviors; callousness is the opposite of prosociality.[44,52,53] Children who are high on dispositional prosociality are helpful and caring and, therefore, evoke mostly positive social behaviors from adults and peers. This promotes the learning of adaptive social skills. In addition, when children who are high in prosociality happen to behave in ways that upset others, the natural consequences of their behaviors are punishing. Seeing that others have been upset by their words or actions makes children who are high in prosociality feel bad. Seeing others upset by their behavior is punishing and guilt inducing, reducing the likelihood of their engaging in such upsetting behaviors in the future. Furthermore, children high in prosociality care about other people and are more responsive to social rewards, fostering the learning of adaptive behavior.[54]

Consider the other end of the prosociality dimension. Children low in prosociality find the adverse consequences of their misbehaviors on others to be neutral or even reinforcing. Consider an example of the hypothesized role played by dispositions in our transactions with the environment. Imagine two 4-year-old girls enrolled in different preschools who are each playing with a toy car. In each preschool, a boy suddenly tries to pull the car away from the girl. In the ensuing tussle over the car, each of our hypothetical girls hits the boy in the nose with the car, making him cry in pain as his nose begins to bleed. Each girl keeps the car when the boy releases it. Now, imagine one of these girls is high in prosociality—that is, she tends to care about the well-being of others and feels guilty when she does something wrong. For this prosocial girl, seeing the boy cry and bleed would likely be very upsetting and would punish her act of physical aggression, making her less likely to be aggressive again.

Antisocial behavior is likely self-punishing in children who are high in prosociality.[55] From this transaction, she would likely learn not to be physically aggressive, giving her the opportunity to learn assertive ways to stand up for herself in nonviolent ways. In contrast, if the other girl is characteristically low in prosociality, she would not be upset by seeing the boy cry. She might even enjoy it! Unfortunately, she may be rewarded by getting the car and learn to use violence to get what she wants.

Thus, exactly the same experience can teach very different things to different people with different dispositional characteristics. Consider that statement for a moment. No two people live in the same world; even if they did, they would not react to the world in the same ways.

Fearful Avoidance versus Daring

Children who are high in fearful avoidance stay clear of risky situations and potential dangers.[56,57] In contrast, persons who are low in fearful avoidance behave in daring ways. They are less likely to avoid harmful situations and often find intense and risky situations to be attractive and rewarding. Thus, the rough-and-tumble of fighting, the intense stimulation of vandalism, and the risk of being caught when shop-lifting are attractive and positively reinforcing to daring children and teach them to be antisocial, whereas these same consequences would likely be punishing to children who are high in fearful avoidance.

Cognitive Abilities

Thus far, I have described dispositions that influence our transactions with the environment that are trait-like aspects of emotional and so-cial behavior. In addition, multiple aspects of our cognitive abilities function as dispositions that increase or decrease our likelihood of developing psychological problems. Several aspects cognitive ability predispose children to externalizing behavior problems. These pre-disposing cognitive characteristics include both language deficits[58,59] and deficiencies in executive functions.[60-62] Executive functions are hypothesized to play an important role in the regulation of atten-tion, impulses, and emotions and are therefore robustly related to many kinds of psychological problems.[13,63-68] Like socioemotional dispositions, individual differences in cognitive abilities influence how we behave, how the world responds to us, and what we learn from the world.

Demographic Differences in Dispositions

Our transactions with our environments are influenced in important ways by our age, sex, and race and ethnicity. Sometimes fairly, but very often unfairly, our social worlds react to us based on our demographic characteristics. To understand this issue by focusing on one example, it will be useful to use the concept of dispositional traits to return to the topic of sex differences for a moment. There are average sex differences in some of the dispositions that influence the transactions of females and males.[69,70] On average—which means that the differences are not true of every girl and boy—girls tend to be more prosocial and fearful and boys tend to be less prosocial and more prone to fearless sensation-seeking. Thus, sex differences in dispositions may play a role in the origins of sex differences in psychological problems. Interestingly, there is no sex difference in negative emotionality.

Transactional Spirals and Stress Generation

When children engage in maladaptive behaviors, those behaviors can understandably change how people respond to them, which can further worsen the children's behavior. A remarkable study of approximately 2,400 girls living in Pittsburgh, Pennsylvania, sheds light on such transactional spirals by assessing the child's disobedient and oppositional behavior and the parent's behavior toward the child annually from kindergarten through high school.[71] From one year to the next, having parents who frequently yelled, threatened, and attempted to verbally coerce their child into obeying predicted increasing levels of child oppositional behavior. In turn, greater child oppositional behavior predicted higher levels of parental verbal aggression in the following year. These difficult daughters made their difficult parents worse, and vice versa, through transactional spirals.

Psychologists Connie Hammen and Lauren Alloy added an exceptionally import element to our understanding of transactional spirals that worsen psychological problems. They offered the *stress generation hypothesis*.[72,73] This hypothesis distinguishes between two types of stressful events—those that occur independently of our behavior, such as earthquakes or all employees being laid off because of the closing of a company, and dependent stressors that at least partly depend on our behavior. Examples of dependent stressors include being fired for poor performance, having a beloved spouse ask for a divorce, or being incarcerated for a crime. Those are dependent stressors because, in each case, the likelihood of their occurrence at least partly depended on the person's actions, such as uncontrolled drinking causing the spouse to ask for a divorce and committing crimes leading to incarceration.

There is increasing evidence that depressed persons generate dependent stressful events for themselves, and those events further predict future depression beyond what would be expected on the basis of their current depression.[73-76] For example, a longitudinal study of several hundred adolescents assessed eight times at 3-month intervals over 2 years revealed a two-way reciprocal relationship between some kinds of stress and depression.[76] Youth who experienced more stressful interpersonal experiences in each assessment reported more depression during the next 3 months. Conversely, youth who reported more depression were more likely to experience interpersonal stressors that were at least partly dependent on their own behavior in the following 3 months.[76]

Depression is not the only kind of psychological problem that can cause stressful events, of course. For example, persons with social anxiety appear to interact with others in ways that generate conflict, rejection, and other kinds of interpersonal stress.[77] Similarly, several studies have confirmed Gerald Patterson's hypothesis that child and adolescent conduct problems cause the stressful events of school expulsions and arrests, which in turn precipitate depression in the youth.[78-81]

Again, the concepts of stress-generation described in this chapter and active and evocative gene-environment correlation discussed in Chapter 8 overlap in meaning. The only differences is that gene-environment correlation is limited to genetically influenced characteristics of the person, whereas stress generation is not. The thrust is the same, however; we often create our own stressful worlds.

Closing Thoughts about Dispositions and Transactions

Dispositions Work Together

I have described some of the evidence that is consistent with the hypothesis that several dispositional traits increase the likelihood of later psychological problems, almost certainly through transactional processes. In addition, there is evidence that these different dispositions *work together* to influence the likelihood of their future psychological problems. My colleagues and I investigated the possibility that extremes on three dispositions in children and adolescents would each predict the problems that define the diagnosis of antisocial personality disorder 12 years later in adulthood.[81] We found that youth self-ratings at ages 10–17 years of their own greater negative emotionality, greater daring, and lower prosociality each significantly predicted an increased likelihood of their adult antisocial behaviors. The contributions of these three dispositional dimensions were independent. This means that the predictive power of each disposition *adds* to the others to jointly predict future antisocial behavior a dozen years later surprisingly well.

Heterogeneity in Psychological Problems

Considering dispositions may well help us understand the *heterogeneity* of psychological problems. By that, I mean that different people who exhibit high levels of the same kinds of psychological problem may do so for different reasons. In the case of adult antisocial behavior, for example, the evidence suggests that some antisocial adults are low in prosociality but have average levels of negative emotionality and daring. Those persons might well have developed adult antisocial behavior for different reasons than equally antisocial adults who are high solely in daring. Many psychologists and psychiatrists believe that this possibility suggests that we should study the causes and neural mechanisms of each of the separate dispositions rather than of heterogeneous antisocial behavior—or depression or schizophrenia, etc.[82]

References

1. Regehr C, Regehr G, Bradford J. A model for predicting depression in victims of rape. *Journal of the American Academy of Psychiatry Law.* 1998;26(4):595–605.

2. Marks NF, Jun H, Song J. Death of parents and adult psychological and physical well-being—A prospective US national study. *Journal of Family Issues.* 2007;28(12):1611–1638.

3. Wikman A, Mattsson E, von Essen L, Hoven E. Prevalence and predictors of symptoms of anxiety and depression, and comorbid symptoms of distress in parents of childhood cancer survivors and bereaved parents five years after end of treatment or a child's death. *Acta Oncologica.* 2018;57(7):950–957.

4. Brent D, Melhem N, Donohoe B. The incidence and course of depression in bereaved youth 21 months after the loss of a parent to suicide, accident, or sudden natural death. *American Journal of Psychiatry.* 2009;166(7):786–794.

5. Porter B, Hoge CW, Tobin LE, et al. Measuring aggregated and specific combat exposures: Associations between combat exposure measures and posttraumatic stress disorder, depression, and alcohol-related problems. *Journal of Traumatic Stress.* 2018;31(2):296–306.

6. Lereya ST, Copeland WE, Costello EJ, Wolke D. Adult mental health consequences of peer bullying and maltreatment in childhood: Two cohorts in two countries. *Lancet Psychiatry.* 2015;2(6):524–531.

7. Stikkelbroek Y, Bodden DHM, Reitz E, Vollebergh WAM, van Baar AL. Mental health of adolescents before and after the death of a parent or sibling. *European Child & Adolescent Psychiatry.* 2016;25(1):49–59.

8. Kingsbury M, Sucha E, Manion I, Gilman SE, Colman I. Adolescent mental health following exposure to positive and harsh parenting in childhood. *Canadian Journal of Psychiatry.* 2020;65(6):392–400.

9. Afifi TO, MacMillan HL, Boyle M, Taillieu T, Cheung K, Sareen J. Child abuse and mental disorders in Canada. *Canadian Medical Association Journal.* 2014;186(9):E324–E332.

10. Schaefer JD, Moffitt TE, Arseneault L, et al. Adolescent victimization and early-adult psychopathology: Approaching causal inference using a longitudinal twin study to rule out noncausal explanations. *Clinical Psychological Science.* 2018;6(3):352–371.

11. Asselmann E, Wittchen HU, Lieb R, Beesdo-Baum K. A 10-year prospective–longitudinal study of daily hassles and incident psychopathology among adolescents and young adults: Interactions with gender, perceived coping efficacy, and negative life events. *Social Psychiatry and Psychiatric Epidemiology.* 2017;52(11):1353–1362.

12. Keles S, Idsoe T, Friborg O, Sirin S, Oppedal B. The longitudinal relation between daily hassles and depressive symptoms among unaccompanied refugees in Norway. *Journal of Abnormal Child Psychology.* 2017;45(7):1413–1427.

13. Bell, R. Q. A reinterpretation of the direction of effects in studies of socialization. *Psychological Review.* 1968;75:81–95.

14. Ebrahimi OV, Hoffart A, Johnson SU. Physical distancing and mental health during the COVID-19 pandemic: Factors associated with psychological symptoms and adherence to pandemic mitigation strategies. *Clinical Psychological Science.* 2021:1–18.

15. Fortgang RG, Wang SB, Millner AJ, et al. Increase in suicidal thinking during COVID-19. *Clinical Psychological Science.* 2021:1–7.

16. Keenan K, Berona J, Hipwell AE, Stepp SD, Romito MT. Validity of the Trier Social Stress Test in studying discrimination stress. *Stress.* 2021;24(1):113–119.

17. Hasin DS, Grant BF. The National Epidemiologic Survey on Alcohol and Related Conditions (NESARC) Waves 1 and 2: Review and summary of findings. *Social Psychiatry and Psychiatric Epidemiology.* 2015;50(11):1609–1640.

18. Network NECCR. Duration and developmental timing of poverty and children's cognitive and social development from birth through third grade. *Child Development.* 2005;76:795–810.

19. Hakulinen C, Webb RT, Pedersen CB, Agerbo E, Mok PLH. Association between parental income during childhood and risk of schizophrenia later in life. *JAMA Psychiatry.* 2020;77:17–24.

20. Kawakami N, Abdulghani EA, Alonso J, et al. Early-life mental disorders and adult household income in the World Mental Health Surveys. *Biological Psychiatry.* 2012;72(3):228–237.

21. Parmar D, Stavropoulou C, Ioannidis JPA. Health outcomes during the 2008 financial crisis in Europe: Systematic literature review. *British Medical Journal.* 2016;354:i4588.

22. Frasquilho D, Matos MG, Salonna F, et al. Mental health outcomes in times of economic recession: A systematic literature review. *BMC Public Health.* 2016;16:115.

23. Forbes MK, Krueger RF. The great recession and mental health in the United States. *Clinical Psychological Science.* 2019;7(5):900–913.

24. Ridley M, Rao G, Schilbach F, Patel V. Poverty, depression, and anxiety: Causal evidence and mechanisms. *Science.* 2020;370:6522.

25. D'Onofrio BM, Goodnight JA, Van Hulle CA, et al. A quasi-experimental analysis of the association between family income and offspring conduct problems. *Journal of Abnormal Child Psychology.* 2009;37:415–429.

26. Costello EJ, Compton SN, Keeler G, Angold A. Relationships between poverty and psychopathology: A natural experiment. *JAMA.* 2003;290:2023–2029.

27. Conger RD, Ge XJ, Elder GH, Lorenz FO, Simons RL. Economic stress, co-ercive family process, and developmental problems of adolescents. *Child Development.* 1994;65:541–561.

28. Generaal E, Hoogendijk EO, Stam M, et al. Neighbourhood char-acteristics and prevalence and severity of depression: Pooled anal-ysis of eight Dutch cohort studies. *British Journal of Psychiatry.* 2019;215(2):468–475.

29. Goodnight JA, Lahey BB, Van Hulle CA, et al. A quasi-experimental anal-ysis of the influence of neighborhood disadvantage on child and adolescent conduct problems. *Journal of Abnormal Psychology.* 2012;121(1):95–108.

30. Belsky DW, Caspi A, Arseneault L, et al. Genetics and the geog-raphy of health, behaviour and attainment. *Nature Human Behaviour.* 2019;3(6):576–586.

31. Curry A, Latkin C, Davey-Rothwell M. Pathways to depression: The im-pact of neighborhood violent crime on inner-city residents in Baltimore, Maryland, USA. *Social Science & Medicine.* 2008;67(1):23–30.

32. Jones AM, Adams RE. Examining the effects of individual-level and neighborhood-level characteristics on the variability of substance use rates and changes. *Journal of Drug Issues.* 2018;48(3):337–355.

33. Mason MJ, Light JM, Mennis J, et al. Neighborhood disorder, peer net-work health, and substance use among young urban adolescents. *Drug and Alcohol Dependence.* 2017;178:208–214.

34. Ludwig J, Duncan GJ, Gennetian LA, et al. Neighborhood effects on the long-term well-being of low-income adults. *Science.* 2012;337(6101):1505–1510.

35. Khan A, Plana-Ripoll O, Antonsen S, et al. Environmental pollution is associated with increased risk of psychiatric disorders in the US and Denmark. *PLoS Biology.* 2019;17(8):e3000353.

36. Newbury JB, Arseneault L, Beevers S, et al. Association of air pollution ex-posure with psychotic experiences during adolescence. *JAMA Psychiatry.* 2019;76(6):614–623.

37. Bandura A. *Principles of behavior modification.* New York, NY: Holt, Rinehart & Winston; 1969.

38. Patterson GR, DeBaryshe BD, Ramsey E. A developmental perspective on antisocial behavior. *American Psychologist.* 1989;44:329–335.

39. Sameroff AJE, ed. *The transactional model of development: How children and contexts shape each other.* Washington, DC: American Psychological Association; 2009.

40. Patterson GR. *Coercive family process.* Eugene, OR: Castalia; 1982.

41. Sameroff A. Transactional models in early social relations. *Human Development.* 1975;18(1–2):65–79.

42. Anderson KE, Lytton H, Romney DM. Mothers' interactions with normal and conduct disordered boys: Who affects whom. *Developmental Psychology.* 1986;22(5):604–609.

43. Mischel W. Toward an integrative science of the person. *Annual Review of Psychology*. 2004;55:1–22.

44. Waldman ID, Tackett JL, Van Hulle CA, et al. Child and adolescent conduct disorder substantially shares genetic influences with three socioemotional dispositions. *Journal of Abnormal Psychology*. 2011;120:57–70.

45. Lahey BB, Krueger RF, Rathouz PJ, Waldman ID, Zald DH. A hierarchical causal taxonomy of psychopathology across the life span. *Psychological Bulletin*. 2017;143:142–186.

46. Servaas MN, van der Velde J, Costafreda SG, et al. Neuroticism and the brain: A quantitative meta-analysis of neuroimaging studies investigating emotion processing. *Neuroscience and Biobehavioral Reviews*. 2013;37(8):1518–1529.

47. Compas BE, Connor-Smith J, Jaser SS. Temperament, stress reactivity, and coping: Implications for depression in childhood and adolescence. *Journal of Clinical Child and Adolescent Psychology*. 2004;33(1):21–31.

48. Jeronimus BF, Kotov R, Riese H, Ormel J. Neuroticism's prospective association with mental disorders halves after adjustment for baseline symptoms and psychiatric history, but the adjusted association hardly decays with time: A meta-analysis on 59 longitudinal/prospective studies with 443,313 participants. *Psychological Medicine*. 2016;46:2883–2906.

49. Brookings JB, Zembar MJ, Hochstetler GM. An interpersonal circumplex/five-factor analysis of the Rejection Sensitivity Questionnaire. *Personality and Individual Differences*. 2003;34(3):449–461.

50. Cain NM, De Panfilis C, Meehan KB, Clarkin JF. A multisurface interpersonal circumplex assessment of rejection sensitivity. *Journal of Personality Assessment*. 2017;99(1):35–45.

51. Snyder J, Reid JB, Patterson GR. A social learning model of child and adolescent antisocial behavior. In: Lahey BB, Moffitt TE, Caspi A, eds. *Causes of conduct disorder and juvenile delinquency*. New York, NY: Guilford; 2003:27–48.

52. Lahey BB. What we need to know about callous-unemotional traits: Comment on Frick, Ray, Thornton, and Kahn (2014). *Psychological Bulletin*. 2014;140:58–63.

53. Frick PJ, Ray JV, Thornton LC, Kahn RE. Can callous-unemotional traits enhance the understanding, diagnosis, and treatment of serious conduct problems in children and adolescents? A comprehensive review. *Psychological Bulletin*. 2014;140:1–57.

54. Lahey BB, Waldman ID. Annual research review: Phenotypic and causal structure of conduct disorder in the broader context of prevalent forms of psychopathology. *Journal of Child Psychology and Psychiatry*. 2012;53:536–557.

55. Frick PJ, Viding E. Antisocial behavior from a developmental psychopathology perspective. *Development and Psychopathology*. 2009;21:1111–1131.

56. Biederman J, Hirshfeld-Becker DR, Rosenbaum JF, et al. Further evidence of association between behavioral inhibition and social anxiety in children. *American Journal of Psychiatry.* 2001;158(10):1673–1679.

57. Schwartz CE, Snidman N, Kagan J. Early childhood temperament as a determinant of externalizing behavior in adolescence. *Development and Psychopathology.* 1996;8(3):527–537.

58. Keenan K, Shaw DS. Starting at the beginning: Exploring the etiology of antisocial behavior in the first years of life. In: Lahey BB, Moffitt TE, Caspi A, eds. *Causes of conduct disorder and juvenile delinquency.* New York, NY: Guilford; 2003:153–181.

59. Lahey BB, D'Onofrio BM, Van Hulle CA, Rathouz PJ. Prospective association of childhood receptive vocabulary and conduct problems with self-reported adolescent delinquency: Tests of mediation and moderation in sibling-comparison analyses. *Journal of Abnormal Child Psychology.* 2014;42:1341–1351.

60. Granvald V, Marciszko C. Relations between key executive functions and aggression in childhood. *Child Neuropsychology.* 2016;22:537–555.

61. Nigg JT, Huang-Pollock CL. An early-onset model of the role of executive functions and intelligence in conduct disorder/delinquency. In: Lahey BB, Moffitt TE, Caspi A, eds. *Causes of conduct disorder and juvenile delinquency.* New York, NY: Guilford; 2003:227–253.

62. Morgan AB, Lilienfeld SO. A meta-analytic review of the relation between antisocial behavior and neuropsychological measures of executive function. *Clinical Psychology Review.* 2000;20:113–136.

63. Grotzinger AD, Cheung AK, Patterson MW, Harden KP, Tucker-Drob EM. Genetic and environmental links between general factors of psychopathology and cognitive ability in early childhood. *Clinical Psychological Science.* 2019;7(3):430–444.

64. Martel MM, Pan PM, Hoffmann MS, et al. A general psychopathology factor (p factor) in children: Structural model analysis and external validation through familial risk and child global executive function. *Journal of Abnormal Psychology.* 2017;126:137–148.

65. Friedman NP, Miyake A. Unity and diversity of executive functions: Individual differences as a window on cognitive structure. *Cortex.* 2017;86:186–204.

66. Hatoum AS, Rhee SH, Corley RP, Hewitt JK, Friedman NP. Do executive functions explain the covariance between internalizing and externalizing behaviors? *Development and Psychopathology.* 2018;30(4):1371–1387.

67. McTeague LM, Goodkind MS, Etkin A. Transdiagnostic impairment of cognitive control in mental illness. *Journal of Psychiatric Research.* 2016;83:37–46.

68. McTeague LM, Huemer J, Carreon DM, Jiang Y, Eickhoff SB, Etkin A. Identification of common neural circuit disruptions in cognitive

control across psychiatric disorders. *American Journal of Psychiatry*. 2017;174(7):676–685.

69. Lahey BB, Applegate B, Chronis AM, et al. Psychometric characteristics of a measure of emotional dispositions developed to test a developmental propensity model of conduct disorder. *Journal of Clinical Child and Adolescent Psychology*. 2008;37:794–807.

70. Lahey BB, Rathouz PJ, Applegate B, Tackett JL, Waldman ID. Psychometrics of a self-report version of the Child and Adolescent Dispositions Scale. *Journal of Clinical Child and Adolescent Psychology*. 2010;39:351–361.

71. Derella OJ, Burke JD, Stepp SD, Hipwell AE. Reciprocity in undesirable parent–child behavior? Verbal aggression, corporal punishment, and girls' oppositional defiant symptoms. *Journal of Clinical Child and Adolescent Psychology*. 2020;49(3):420–433.

72. Hammen C. Stress generation in depression: Reflections on origins, research, and future directions. *Journal of Clinical Psychology*. 2006;62(9):1065–1082.

73. Alloy LB, Liu RT, Bender RE. Stress generation research in depression: A commentary. *International Journal of Cognitive Therapy*. 2010;3(4):380–388.

74. Kendler KS, Gardner CO. Dependent stressful life events and prior depressive episodes in the prediction of major depression. *Archives of General Psychiatry*. 2010;67(11):1120–1127.

75. Snyder HR, Friedman NP, Hankin BL. Transdiagnostic mechanisms of psychopathology in youth: Executive functions, dependent stress, and rumination. *Cognitive Therapy and Research*. 2019;43(5):834–851.

76. Jenness JL, Peverill M, King KM, Hankin BL, McLaughlin KA. Dynamic associations between stressful life events and adolescent internalizing psychopathology in a multiwave longitudinal study. *Journal of Abnormal Psychology*. 2019;128(6):596–609.

77. Siegel DM, Burke TA, Hamilton JL, Piccirillo ML, Scharff A, Alloy LB. Social anxiety and interpersonal stress generation: The moderating role of interpersonal distress. *Anxiety Stress and Coping*. 2018;31(5):526–538.

78. Patterson GR, Capaldi DM. A mediational model for boys' depressed mood. In: Rolf JE, ed. *Risk and protective factors in the development of psychopathology*. New York, NY: Cambridge University Press; 1990:141–163.

79. Patterson GR, Stoolmiller M. Replications of a dual failure model for boys' depressed mood. *Journal of Consulting and Clinical Psychology*. 1991;59:491–498.

80. Burke JD, Loeber R, Lahey BB, Rathouz PJ. Developmental transitions among affective and behavioral disorders in adolescent boys. *Journal of Child Psychology and Psychiatry*. 2005;46:1200–1210.

81. Lahey BB, Class QA, Zald DH, Rathouz PJ, Applegate B, Waldman ID. Prospective test of the developmental propensity model of antisocial behavior: From childhood and adolescence into early adulthood. *Journal of Child Psychology and Psychiatry*. 2018;59:676–683.

82. Cuthbert BN, Insel TR. Toward the future of psychiatric diagnosis: The seven pillars of RDoC. *BMC Medicine*. 2013;11:126.

Epilogue

In this book, I have joined with other psychologists and psychiatrists[1-4] to advocate a *positive revolution* in our understanding of psychological problems. This revolution will require leaving behind the untenable medical model of binary diagnostic categories that is the basis of the *Diagnostic and Statistical Manual of Mental Disorders* (DSM) and replacing it with an entirely dimensional model of psychological problems. Some of the ideas that undergird this revolution have been around for many years, and others reflect new understandings of psychological problems that recent data have allowed us to see. I argue here for a new view of psychological problems that is far less stigmatizing and much better supported by the data. This revolution will require several related changes in thinking:

- There is no qualitative difference between "normal" and "abnormal" psychological functioning. Psychological problems do not reflect rare and terrifying "illnesses" of the mind. Rather, psychological problems are simply problematic ways of thinking, feeling, and behaving that lie on continuous dimensions from minor to severe.
- There are no clear boundaries among the various dimensions of psychological problems. Rather, the dimensions are highly correlated and overlapping. This means that people often experience psychological problems from more than one dimension at the same time.
- Crucially, psychological problems are *ordinary* aspects of the human experience. This is true in two important ways. First, longitudinal studies of the general population have revealed that the great majority of us will experience distressing and disruptive psychological problems at some time during our lives. Second,

psychological problems arise through the same natural and ordinary processes as do all aspects of behavior.

- The patterns of correlations among the various dimensions of psychological problems provide vital clues to the causes of psychological problems. These correlations reflect a hierarchy ranging from nonspecific causes—that influence the likelihood of exhibiting *some* kind of psychological problems, but not *which* ones—to increasingly more specific causes that influence which particular problems will be exhibited. Research based on this view of a hierarchy of causal influences has already been informative and should continue to advance our understanding of the origins of psychological problems.[4-6]

- Although there is some stability in psychological problems over time, they change over the course of our lives. Importantly, these patterns of developmental change are often substantially different for females and males. We will not achieve a comprehensive understanding of psychological problems until we understand the causes of sex differences in prevalence, incidence, and developmental change.

- Adaptive and maladaptive patterns of behavior arise through the same natural interplay of genes and environments. This occurs during transactions with the environment in which heritable aspects of the person's behavior are influenced by the environment, and the person's behavior also both influences the environment and helps determine how the person will respond to the environment.

Like others, I argue that this model of correlated dimensions of psychological problems can and should replace the stigma-laden diagnostic categories of DSM and help people understand their psychological problems as far less threatening natural phenomena. Furthermore, framing psychological problems as hierarchically correlated dimensions should lead to more informative research on causes and mechanisms compared to the untenable model of distinct mental disorders with different causes and mechanisms. A focus on heritable dispositional constructs that play key roles in transactions should help us understand the causal and mechanistic heterogeneity of each dimension of psychological problems. This, in turn, should inform and support tests of new methods of prevention and intervention.

References

1. Clark LA, Watson D, Reynolds S. Diagnosis and classification of psychopathology: Challenges to the current system and future directions. *Annual Review of Psychology.* 1995;46:121–153.
2. Kotov R, Krueger RF, Watson D, et al. The Hierarchical Taxonomy of Psychopathology (HiTOP): A dimensional alternative to traditional nosologies. *Journal of Abnormal Psychology.* 2017;126(4):454–477.
3. Krueger RF, Markon KE. A dimensional-spectrum model of psychopathology: Progress and opportunities. *Archives of General Psychiatry.* 2011;68:10–11.
4. Lahey BB, Krueger RF, Rathouz PJ, Waldman ID, Zald DH. A hierarchical causal taxonomy of psychopathology across the life span. *Psychological Bulletin.* 2017;143:142–186.
5. Kaczkurkin AN, Moore TM, Sotiras A, Xia CH, Shinohara RT, Satterthwaite TD. Approaches to defining common and dissociable neurobiological deficits associated with psychopathology in youth. *Biological Psychiatry.* 2020;88(1):51–62.
6. Smoller JW, Andreassen OA, Edenberg HJ, Faraone SV, Glatt SJ, Kendler KS. Psychiatric genetics and the structure of psychopathology. *Molecular Psychiatry.* 2019;24(3):409–420.

Technical Appendix

Factor Analysis

Factor analysis is a statistical method that is frequently used by researchers to help define dimensions of psychological problems (and second-order factors). A matrix of every possible correlation among a set of each quantitatively measured psychological problem is first calculated. For example, each specific psychological problem (uncontrollable worry, irritability, grandiose self-esteem, etc.) might be rated on its frequency and severity on a scale from 0 to 3. Then, those ratings of every specific problem are correlated with one another in a sample of, for example, 1,000 people. It is common to find that some subsets of psychological problems are more correlated among themselves than they are with other problems.

I illustrate this visually. In Figure A.1, each dot represents a different specific psychological problem. The black and white dots represent two subgroups of such specific psychological problems. The lengths of the lines connecting the black dots represent the magnitudes of the correlations among them. Dots that are closer together in this figure are more strongly correlated. This just means that if the raters of the 1,000 people give a higher rating to one problem represented by a black dot, they will tend to give a higher rating to other problems represented by black dots that are nearby. Thus, the black dots

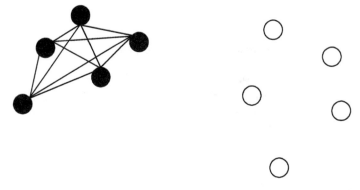

Figure A.1

represent problems that are substantially correlated with one another. The same is true for the set of white dots. Therefore, the black dots and the white dots represent two sets of correlated problems. Note that the white dots are not far from the black dots. Nonetheless, the black dots and white dots are correlated with one another (lines not shown), but the black and white dots are less correlated than the dots of the same color are correlated with one another.

Factor scores for each person on black problems and factor scores for white problems can be calculated. In theory, the measures black problems hang together because each set of tightly correlated black problems is a manifestation of an unmeasured "factor" that causes the problems to be correlated. That factor can be estimated mathematically from the matrix of correlations in factor analysis (illustrated by the gray square in Figure A.2).

To make this illustration more concrete, assume that the correlated problems are the "symptoms" of two "mental disorders" that are sometimes observed in adolescents—conduct disorder and depression (Figure A.3). The

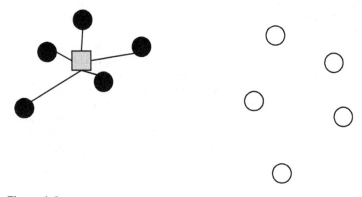

Figure A.2

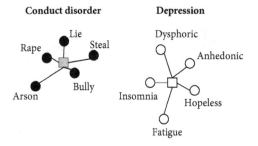

Figure A.3

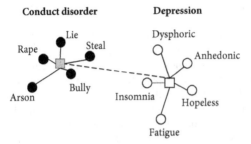

Figure A.4

gray and white squares presented are the mathematically estimated first-order factor scores for each person on these two factors of psychological problems. When dimensions of psychological problems are measured, such factor scores are used to quantify the dimensions instead of simply summing ratings of the individual items.

It is possible to calculate the correlation between these two factor scores (illustrated by the dotted line in Figure A.4). When this has been done for many different sets of specific psychological problems, every dimension based on factors of psychological problems has been found to be positively correlated in large samples that represent the population. When I say that every dimension of psychological problems is positively correlated with every other dimension, I mean that the factor scores are more positively correlated with one another than would be expected by chance.

Reliability of DSM-5 Diagnoses

The Task Force of the American Psychiatric Association that developed the fifth edition of the *Diagnostic and Statistical Manual of Mental Disorders* (DSM-5) conducted a field trial using a number of institutions in the United States and Canada to evaluate the test–retest reliability of the most commonly used DSM-5 diagnostic categories. A total of 279 clinicians were trained in DSM-5 criteria and then asked to conduct independent diagnostic assessments a few hours up to 14 days later of about 2,000 persons enrolled in mental health clinics. In simple terms, they examined the extent to which the two interviewers gave the same diagnosis. They used a standard metric of test–retest agreement, called Cohen's kappa,[1] that adjusts for chance agreements. That is, even two computers who were randomly giving the diagnosis of X would both say "X" some of the time and both say "not X" some of the time by chance. Cohen's kappa calculates the percentage agreement on the presence and absence of diagnosis X, above and beyond such chance agreements.[1] By convention, a kappa coefficient of 0.40 or greater is considered to reflect an acceptable level of agreement.

In the DSM-5 field trials, some important kinds of psychological problems were diagnosed with acceptable reliability, including schizophrenia, bipolar disorder, and post-traumatic stress disorder, but a surprising 40% of diagnoses examined did not reach the 0.40 cutoff for acceptable interrater agreement.[2] Shockingly, the test–retest reliability of the diagnosis of major depressive disorder was considerably below this level at kappa = 0.28, and the reliability of generalized anxiety disorder was even lower at kappa = 0.20. Major depression and generalized anxiety disorder are very common among persons seeking psychiatric help, and diagnosing these mental disorders is the bread-and-butter of psychiatric practice. If everything we believe about psychiatric diagnosis is sensible, these straightforward problems should be diagnosed with high reliability, but the two interviewers agreed on these diagnoses at barely above chance levels.

Furthermore, among the diagnoses that did reach the threshold for acceptable test–retest reliability, the common and important diagnosis of alcohol use disorder was barely acceptable at a level of kappa = 0.40. Because the concrete meaning of Cohen's kappa will not be familiar to most readers, I created a table of agreement between two hypothetical interviewers for the diagnosis of X, which stands for any particular diagnosis in this illustration. My goal is to let readers see how much agreement among interviewers constitutes a Cohen's kappa of 0.40. In the hypothetical illustration in Figure A.5, interviewer 1 gave the diagnosis of X to 25/50 = 50% of cases, denoted in the horizontal gray bar. Interviewer 2 gave the diagnosis of X to 30/50 = 60% of cases, denoted in the vertical gray bar. The two interviewers agreed on the presence of diagnosis X in 20 cases and agreed on the absence of diagnosis X in 15 cases, for 70% total agreement. That sounds pretty good until we take chance agreement into account. In the hypothetical table, we would expect the interviewers to agree

Agreement between two interviewers on a mental disorder diagnosis in 50 Hypothetical persons interviewed at a clinic.

| | | Interviewer 2 | | |
		YES	No	Totals
Interviewer 1	YES	**20**	5	25
	No	10	**15**	25
	Totals	30	20	50

Figure A.5

50% of the time by chance, which is only a little less than the actual observed agreement on the diagnosis of X. Expected chance agreement is calculated from the frequency that each interviewer gives the diagnosis of X. In the figure, the percentage chance agreement on the presence of diagnosis X is based on interviewer 1 giving the diagnosis half of the time and interviewer 2 giving the diagnosis 60% of the time (50% × 60% = 30% expected chance agreement on the diagnosis of X). Similarly, the percentage agreement on the absence of X expected by chance would be 50% × 40% = 20%, which means that the total percentage agreement expected by chance would be 30% + 20% = 50%. Cohen's kappa = 70% observed agreement minus the 50% expected chance agreement (70% – 50% = 20%) over the maximum possible improved agreement through reliable diagnosis of (100% – chance agreement of 50%), which is 0.40.

In one-third of the cases given the diagnosis of X by interviewer 1, interviewer 2 disagreed, and in 40% of the cases that interviewer 1 said did not meet criteria for diagnosis, interviewer 2 said that the person did meet criteria for X. Thus, even modest levels of test–retest agreement on a diagnosis that is better than chance reach the conventional cutoff kappa = 0.40, raising concerns about this lenient cutoff.

References

1. Cohen J. A coefficient of agreement for nominal scales. *Educational and Psychological Measurement.* 1960;20(1):37–46.
2. Regier DA, Narrow WE, Clarke DE, et al. DSM-5 field trials in the United States and Canada, Part II: Test–retest reliability of selected categorical diagnoses. *American Journal of Psychiatry.* 2013;170:59–70.

Index

For the benefit of digital users, indexed terms that span two pages (e.g., 52–53) may, on occasion, appear on only one of those pages.

Figures are indicated by f following the page number

abnormal behavior
  definition of, 5
  discontinuing use of term, 10
adaptive behavior
  fostering in children, 202
  lack of threshold with
    psychological problems, 6
  natural processes causing, 9
  psychoactive substance use
    and, 82
  role of fit with environment, 9–10
adolescence
  changes in psychological problems
    during, 141–43
  externalizing problems, 143–45
  internalizing problems, 143
  psychotic and other problems of
    thought and emotion, 145–46
adulthood
  overview of development, 147–48
  psychological problems
    during, 146–47
age differences, 149–51
age of onset, 138
alcohol dependence, 85–86
Alloy, Lauren, 205
anhedonia, 102
anorexic eating problems, 108–9
antisocial behavior. See oppositional
    and antisocial behavior

attention-deficit/hyperactivity
    disorder (ADHD)
  changes in over time, 149–50
  DSM-based diagnosis of, 69
  hyperactivity-impulsivity, 71
  impairment associated with
    ADHD problems, 71–73
  inattention, 69–70
  unwarranted diagnoses of, 35–36
autism spectrum problems
  autistic rigidity and repetitive
    behavior, 107
  autistic spectrum social
    problems, 107–8
  in childhood, 140–41

Bandura, Albert, 5, 7, 10, 19
Bell, Robert, 195–96
binary diagnostic approach
  cross-cutting issues, 46–47
  describing dimensions of
    psychological problems,
    41–46, 43f
  versus dimensional model, 37–41
  overview of, 29–30
  problems of binary
    approach, 30–36
binge eating, 109
borderline emotional
    instability, 64–65

brain abnormalities/dysfunction
associated with exposure to THC
during pregnancy, 87–88
due to immune activation during
pregnancy, 22–23
stigma fostered by perception
of, 19–20
bulimic eating problems, 108–9

cannabis abuse and
dependence, 87–88
Caspi, Avshalon, 118
catatonic behavior, 100–1
causal hypothesis
dimension-specific causal
influences, 126–27
direct and indirect sharing of
causal influences, 127–28
hierarchy of causes, 121–22
highly nonspecific causal
influences, 122f, 122–25
partially nonspecific causal
influences, 125–26
reasons for multiple psychological
problems, 128–30
childhood
autism spectrum
problems, 140–41
changes in psychological problems
during, 139
externalizing problems, 139–40
internalizing problems, 140
cocaine dependence, 86
Cohen's kappa, 35, 221–22
compulsive rigidity and
perfectionism, 106
conversion somatic problems, 110
correlated dimensions, 43f, 43–46,
113, 117, 119. See also
hierarchy of correlations
cross-sectional studies, 135–36

DeFries, John, 171
delusions, 99–100

depersonalization, 96–97
depression, 59–60
derealization, 96–97
detachment, 101
diagnoses
binary diagnostic approach
cross-cutting issues, 46–47
describing dimensions of
psychological problems,
41–46, 43f
versus dimensional
model, 37–41
overview of, 29–30
problems of, 30–34
differential diagnosis, 40
reliability of DSM-5, 35–36,
221–23
Diagnostic and Statistical Manual of
Mental Disorders (DSM-5)
argument for replacement with
dimensional model, xvi–
xviii, 1–2, 4–5, 216–17
author's contributions
toward, 4–5
binary diagnostic categories used
in, xvi–xvii, 215
categorical diagnoses in, 95–
96, 96f
criticisms of, 20
DSM model of psychological
problems, 3–5
polythetic categories in, 32–34
reliability of diagnoses based on,
35, 221–23, 222f
See also diagnoses
differential diagnosis, 40
differentiation, 128–30
dimensional model of psychological
problems
benefits of, 4
binary versus dimensional
approach
benefits of dimensional
model, 37–41

cross-cutting issues, 46–47
describing dimensions of
    psychological problems,
    41–46, 43f
overview of, 29–30
problems of binary
    approach, 30–36
externalizing problems
inattention and hyperactivity-
    impulsivity, 69–73
narcissistic-histrionic
    problems, 82
oppositional and antisocial
    behavior, 73–81
overview of, 68
psychoactive substance use
    problems, 82–88
internalizing problems
borderline emotional
    instability, 64–65
fears and panic attacks, 54–57
overview of, 53–54
social anxiety and
    dependence, 62–64
worry-misery
    problems, 57–62
key aspects of
importance of psychological
    problems, 13–14
ordinariness of psychological
    problems, 9–13
overview of, 5–8
social conflict and
    psychological problems, 8
psychotic and thought/affect
    problems
anorexic and bulimic eating
    problems, 108–9
autistic spectrum
    problems, 106–8
conversion somatic
    problems, 110
dissociative problems, 96–97
manic problems, 103–4

obsessive-compulsive
    problems, 104–6
overview of, 95–96, 96f
psychotic problems, 97–101
schizoid problems, 101–3
as replacement for DSM
    diagnostic categories, xvi–
    xviii, 1–2, 4–5, 216–17
disorganized thinking and
    speech, 100–1
dispositions
cognitive abilities and, 203–4
demographic differences
    in, 204
dispositions work together, 206
fearful avoidance versus
    daring, 203
heterogeneity in psychological
    problems, 206
negative emotionality versus
    emotional stability, 200–2
prosociality versus
    callousness, 202–3
transactional spirals and stress
    generation, 204–5
and transactions, 198–200
dissociative problems, 96–97
DSM-5. See Diagnostic and Statistical
    Manual of Mental Disorders
dynamic development. See sex
    differences and dynamic
    development

early adulthood. See adolescence
economic loss, 13
environmental influences
learning, 194–95
reactions to stress, 194
See also genetic-environmental
    interplay; transactional
    approach
epigenetic modifications, 178–79
evocative gene–environment
    correlation, 172–73

externalizing problems
  in adolescence, 143–45
  in childhood, 139–40
  inattention and hyperactivity-
    impulsivity, 69–73
  narcissistic-histrionic
    problems, 82
  oppositional and antisocial
    behavior, 73–81
  overview of, 43f, 43–46, 68
  psychoactive substance use
    problems, 82–88

factor analysis, 219f, 219–21,
    220f, 221f
fears
  agoraphobic fears, 55–56
  rational versus irrational, 54
  specific fears, 55
first-order dimensions, 115–17
flat affect, 102
Frances, Alan, 20–21

general factor hypothesis
  causal hierarchy hypothesis, 121–
    27, 122f
  direct and indirect sharing of
    causal influences, 127–28
  psychological nature of, 120–21
general factor of intelligence, 118
generalized anxiety, 57–58
general paresis, 2–3
genetic-environmental interplay
  basic gene biology and inheritance
    genetics primer, 164–66
    heritability, 166–70
    pleiotropy and correlated
      dimensions of psychological
      problems, 170–71
  interplay of genes and
    environments
    environments that contribute
      to psychological
      problems, 182–83

gene-environment
    correlation, 172–75
gene-environment
    interactions, 175–81
  heritability and two kinds of
    environments, 181–82
  influence of genes and
    environments, 171
  overview of, 164, 216
  See also environmental influences;
    transactional approach
genetic retrotransposition, 180–81
grandiose beliefs, 100

hallucinations, 99
Halperin, Jeff, 149–50
Hammen, Connie, 205
Haslam, Nick, 19–20
health worries, 58–59
hebephrenic behavior, 100–1
heritability, 166–70, 174
heroin and opioid dependence, 86
heterotypic continuity, 142–43
hierarchy of causes, 121–22, 122f
hierarchy of correlations
  hierarchy of psychological
    problems
    correlated second-order
      dimensions, 117
    first- and second-order
      dimensions, 115–17
    general factor of psychological
      problems, 117–19, 120f
  overview of, 113–15, 115f
  psychological nature of the
    general factor hypothesis
    causal hierarchy hypothesis,
      121–27, 122f
    direct and indirect sharing of
      causal influences, 127–28
    need for further research, 120–21
    reasons for multiple
      psychological
      problems, 128–30

high-risk environments
    confounded by other factors, 188
    discrimination, 190
    disorganized
        neighborhoods, 192–93
    economic hardship, 190–92
    polluted and diminished physical
        environments, 193
    stressful experiences, 189–90
Hinshaw, Steven, 9–10, 20
histrionic-narcissistic problems, 82
hyperactivity-impulsivity, 71

ICD. *See International Classification*
    of Diseases
ideas of reference, 99
impoverished speech, 101
impoverished volition, 101
inattention and
        hyperactivity-impulsivity
    hyperactivity-impulsivity, 71
    impairment associated with
        ADHD problems, 71–73
    inattention, 69–70
incidence, 138, 216
infections
    causing severe psychological
        problems, 2–3
    during pregnancy leading to
        schizophrenic behavior in
        children, 23
internalizing problems
    in adolescence, 143
    borderline emotional
        instability, 64–65
    in childhood, 140
    fears and panic attacks, 54–57
    overview of, 43*f*, 43–46, 53–54
    social anxiety and
        dependence, 62–64
    worry-misery problems, 57–62
International Classification of
    Diseases (ICD)
    adoption of dimensions, 45

binary diagnostic categories used
    in, xvi–xvii

Jones, Ernest, 118, 120–21

Krafft-Ebing, Richard, 2–3
Kvalle, Erlender, 19–20

Lamarck, Jean Baptiste, 179–80
learning, 194–95
Loehlin, John, 171
longevity, reduced expectations for,
    13–14, 83
longitudinal studies, 135–36
Lytton, Hugh, 196

manic problems, 103–4
medical model of psychological
        problems, 2–3, 4–5,
        15, 18–20
mental disorders/mental illness,
    1–5, 15
microglia, 23
mind-body monism, 18–23
model of correlated dimensions.
        See dimensional model of
        psychological problems
Moffitt, Terrie, 118

narcissistic-histrionic problems, 82
neuronal pruning, 22–23
nicotine dependence, 85
nonshared environments, 181

obsessive-compulsive problems
    compulsive rigidity and
        perfectionism, 106
    obsessive-compulsive
        rituals, 104–6
odd beliefs and delusions, 99–100
opioid dependence, 86
oppositional and antisocial behavior
    antisocial behavior and
        gangs, 76–77

oppositional and antisocial
    behavior (*cont.*)
  distressed caused by, 73
  DSM diagnostic categories
    associated with, 80–81
  lack of full understanding
    of, 73–74
  oppositional-defiant
    behavior, 74–75
  proactive antisocial behavior, 76
  psychopathic behavior, 77–80
  reactive antisocial behavior, 75–76
oppositional-defiant behavior, 74–75
ordinary origins of psychological
    problems
  environmental influences
    demographic differences in
      dispositions, 204–6
    environments, 187–95
    overview of, 187
    personal characteristics and
      transactions, 197–204
    transactions with
      environments, 195–97
  genetic-environmental interplay
    basic gene biology and
      inheritance, 164–71
    interplay of genes and
      environments, 171–83
    overview of, 164
  key aspects
    ordinary versus minor, 9
    problems are collectively very
      common, 10–13
    problems are common but
      important, 13–14
    problems arise in ordinary
      ways, 9–10

panic attacks, 56–57
paranoid delusions, 99–100
passive gene–environment
    correlation, 172

Patterson, Gerald, 195–96
perfectionism, 106
pleiotropy, 170–71
Plomin, Robert, 171
political dissidents, 8
polygenic risk scores, 169–70
polythetic categories, 32–34
post-traumatic stress
    reactions, 60–62
prevalence, 138, 216
proactive antisocial behavior, 76
problems in living, 5
Procrustean beds, 31–32
psychiatric medications
  prescribed by inadequately trained
    professionals, 35–36
  unwarranted prescription of, 95
psychoactive substance use problems
  alcohol dependence, 85–86
  cannabis abuse and
    dependence, 87–88
  cocaine dependence, 86
  harm resulting from substance
    abuse, 82–84
  heroin and opioid dependence, 86
  nicotine dependence, 85
  substance abuse and
    dependence, 84–85
psychological help
  accurately describing your
    experience when seeking, 95
  complicated and ethical balancing
    act involved in, 16–18
  deciding to seek help, 6–7
  inherently binary decisions to
    treat or not treat, 12–14
  seeking due to distress based on
    social conflict, 8
psychological problems
  conceptualizing
    DSM model of psychological
      problems, 3–5
    mind-body monism, 18–23

new model of psychological
problems, 5–14
overview of, 1–3
stigma and psychological
problems, 14–18
definition of, 5–6
hierarchical nature of
hierarchy of psychological
problems, 115–19, 120f
overview of, 113–15, 115f
psychological nature of the
general factor hypothesis,
120–30, 122f
positive revolution in
understanding of, xv–
xvii, 215–17
sex differences and dynamic
development of
causes of sex and age
differences, 149–54
overview of, 135–37
psychological problems across
our lives, 137–48
See also dimensional model of
psychological problems;
ordinary origins of
psychological problems
psychopathic behavior, 77–80
psychotic and thought/affect
problems
in adolescence, 145–46
anorexic and bulimic eating
problems, 108–9
autistic spectrum
problems, 106–8
conversion somatic problems, 110
dissociative problems, 96–97
manic problems, 103–4
obsessive-compulsive
problems, 104–6
overview of, 95–96, 96f
psychotic problems, 97–101
schizoid problems, 101–3

reactive antisocial behavior, 75–76
rejection sensitivity, 62–63

Sameroff, Arnold, 195–96
Saving Normal (Frances), 20–21
Schulz, Kurt, 149–50
second-order dimensions, 43f, 43–
44, 115–17
selective gene–environment
correlation, 173
separation anxiety, 63–64
sex differences and dynamic
development
causes of sex and age differences
causes of age
differences, 149–51
causes of sex differences, 151–54
overview of, 135–37
psychological problems across
our lives
adulthood, 146–47
childhood, 139–41
incidence, prevalence, and age
of onset, 138
overview of development, 147–48
transition to adulthood, 141–46
relationship to prevalence,
incidence, and
developmental change, 216
shared causes, 122–27
shared environments, 181
single nucleotide polymorphisms
(SNPs), 165–66
sluggish cognitive tempo, 60
SNPs. See single nucleotide
polymorphisms
social anxiety and dependence,
6, 62–64
social conflict, 8
social dependence, 63–64
social disinterest, 101
somatic delusions, 100
Spearman, Charles, 118

speech, disorganized, 100–1
stigma reduction
    harm resulting from stigma, 14–18
    medical model of psychological
        problems and, 19–20
    preventing discrimination and
        maltreatment, 8
    through new view of psychological
        problems, xvii–xviii, 215
stress generation hypothesis, 205
substance abuse and
        dependence, 84–85
subthreshold symptoms, 12, 38–39
Sullivan, Harry Stack, 5
Szasz, Thomas, 5

test–retest agreement, 35–36, 221–23
thinking, disorganized, 100–1
thought/affect problems. See
        psychotic and thought/affect
        problems
transactional approach
    definition of transactions, 9
    demographic differences in
        dispositions
        dispositions work together, 206
        heterogeneity in psychological
            problems, 206
        transactional spirals and stress
            generation, 204–5

environments
    high-risk, 188–93
    influences on psychological
        problems, 193–95
    overview of, 187
    personal characteristics and
        transactions
        dispositions and transactions,
            198–204
        interactions with the
            world, 197–98
        transactions with environments,
            9–10, 195–97
        See also genetic-environmental
            interplay
transcription, 178
transition to adulthood. See
        adolescence
twin studies, 166–70
typhoid infections, 2–3

worry-misery problems
    depression, 59–60
    generalized anxiety, 57–58
    health worries, 58–59
    post-traumatic stress
        reactions, 60–62
    sluggish cognitive tempo, 60

young adults. See adolescence